My love and thanks to my wonderful family

LEIGH LAWSON

My darling husband, who is the most supportive and loving person in the world.

CARLY LAWSON

My gorgeous daughter, always there for me, and always encouraging. Thank you for your love and support.

JASON LAWSON

My wonderful inherited son, who calls me his 'wicked' stepmother! Thank you for your love and support.

Also my lovely sisters, SHIRLEY and VIVIEN. Growing up with two fashion-conscious, stylish older sisters was probably my first awareness of my passion for fashion.

A Guide to Looking and Feeling Fabulous Over Forty

TWIGGY

with Jenny Dyson

Photography by Brian Aris and Sarah Maingot

Illustrations by Tina Berning

MICHAEL JOSEPH
an imprint of PENGUIN BOOKS

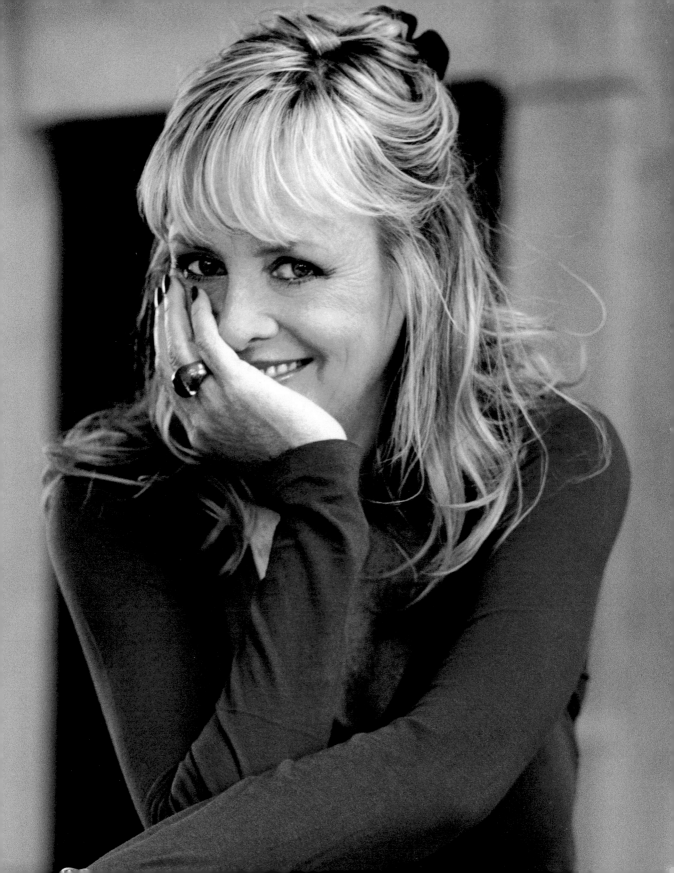

MICHAEL JOSEPH

Published by the Penguin Group

Penguin Books Ltd, 80 Strand, London WC2R 0RL, England

Penguin Group (USA) Inc., 375 Hudson Street, New York, New York 10014, USA

Penguin Group (Canada), 90 Eglinton Avenue East, Suite 700, Toronto, Ontario, Canada M4P 2Y3

(a division of Pearson Penguin Canada Inc.)

Penguin Ireland, 25 St Stephen's Green, Dublin 2, Ireland (a division of Penguin Books Ltd)

Penguin Group (Australia), 250 Camberwell Road,

Camberwell, Victoria 3124, Australia (a division of Pearson Australia Group Pty Ltd)

Penguin Books India Pvt Ltd, 11 Community Centre,

Panchsheel Park, New Delhi – 110 017, India

Penguin Group (NZ), 67 Apollo Drive, Rosedale, North Shore 0632, New Zealand

(a division of Pearson New Zealand Ltd)

Penguin Books (South Africa) (Pty) Ltd, 24 Sturdee Avenue,

Rosebank, Johannesburg 2196, South Africa

Penguin Books Ltd, Registered Offices: 80 Strand, London WC2R 0RL, England

www.penguin.com

First published 2008

1

Text copyright © Twiggy Lawson, 2008

Photography copyright © Brian Aris, 2008, © Benoît Audureau, 2008, © Sarah Maingot, 2008.

Illustrations copyright © Tina Berning, 2008

Art direction and design by Nikki Dupin

The moral right of the author, illustrator and photographers has been asserted

Printed and bound in Italy by Graphicom, srl

Colour reproduction by Altaimage Ltd, UK

A CIP catalogue record for this book is available from the British Library

ISBN: 978–0–718–15404–2

PUBLISHER'S NOTE

Every effort has been made to ensure that the information contained in this book is complete and accurate.
However, neither the publisher nor the author is engaged in rendering professional advice or services to the individual reader.
The ideas, procedures and suggestions contained in this book are not intended as a substitute for consulting with an expert.
All matters regarding your health require medical supervision. Neither the author nor the publisher shall be liable or
responsible for any loss or damage allegedly arising from any information or suggestion in this book.

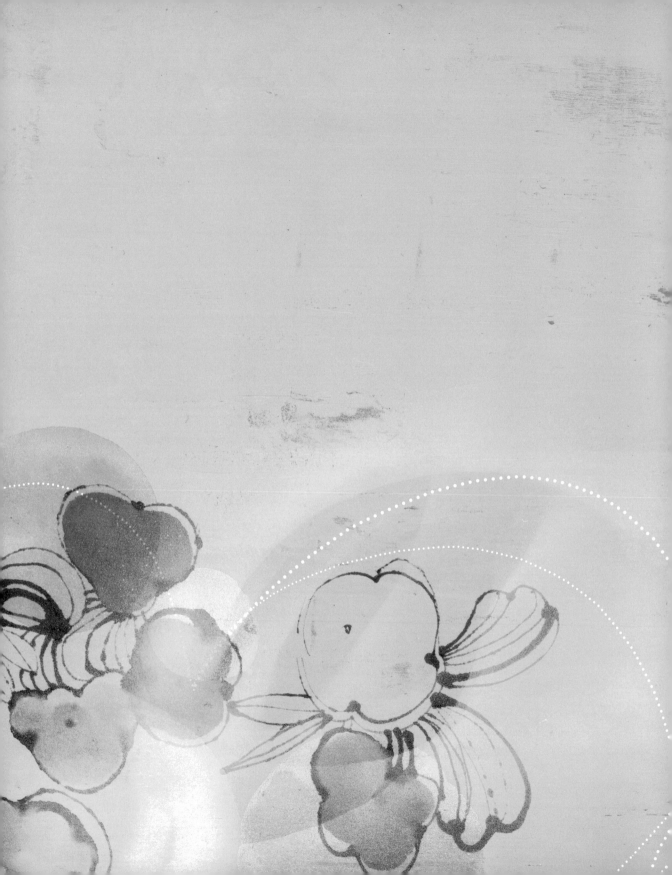

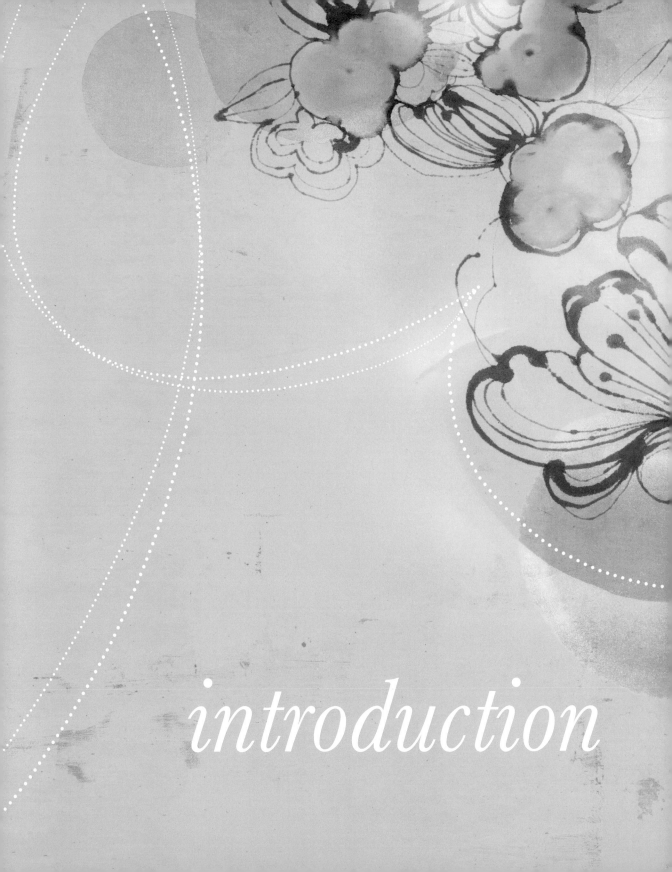

introduction

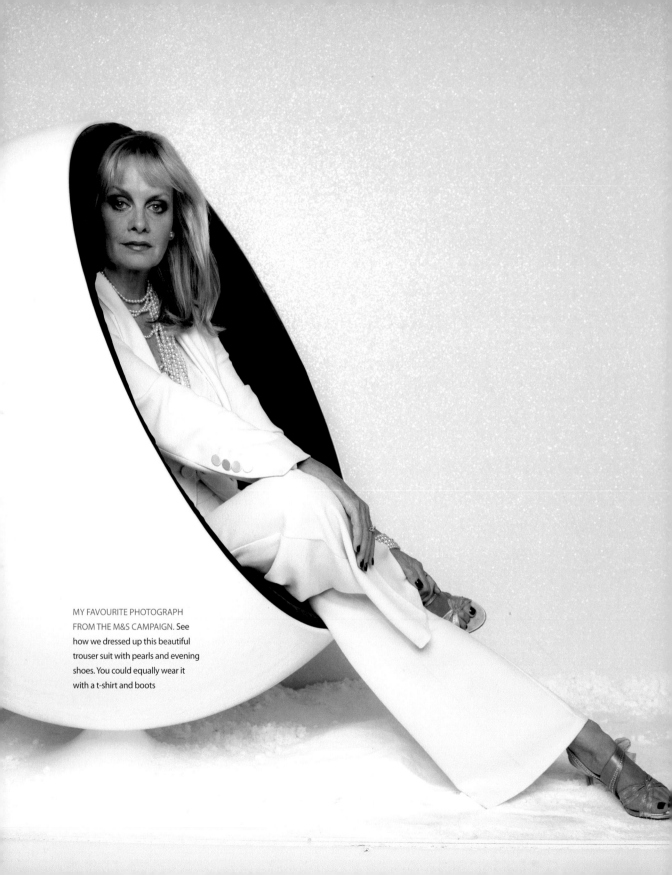

MY FAVOURITE PHOTOGRAPH
FROM THE M&S CAMPAIGN. See
how we dressed up this beautiful
trouser suit with pearls and evening
shoes. You could equally wear it
with a t-shirt and boots

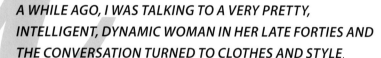

A WHILE AGO, I WAS TALKING TO A VERY PRETTY, INTELLIGENT, DYNAMIC WOMAN IN HER LATE FORTIES AND THE CONVERSATION TURNED TO CLOTHES AND STYLE. She said that she had lost her way with fashion and her self-image had become blurred. 'I don't want to look like mutton dressed as lamb, but I don't want to look like an old frump either,' she said. She then told me a lot of her friends felt the same way.

Crossing the middle-age threshold doesn't mean you have to get out your comfy slippers and your flannel knickers. On the other hand, you really don't want to be flashing the wrong bits. For me, getting older doesn't mean throwing away a favourite coloured lipstick or a fabulous pair of boots; instead it's about harnessing all the great things I have learned over the years about what does and doesn't suit me, and enjoying the way in which cleverly selected outfits can enhance the nice bits. But fashion is easier said than done. In a society where youth is the ultimate obsession, where does that honestly leave us grown-ups? It wasn't so long ago that teenage models were hired to promote anti-wrinkle creams. Thankfully, times are changing.

The forties onwards are when we can really begin to enjoy ourselves. For many women, reaching the fabulous forties and fifties is when everything comes together, and they look better than ever. At this stage of our lives, it's okay to start dedicating a little more time to overall maintenance. Invest any extra time you can spare to beauty and body MOTs and it will pay dividends. Whether it's using experts for a monthly facial, a manicure, pedicure, massage and a regular slot with the hairdresser, or generally taking a little more time to get ready, this added focus on you may feel overindulgent, but it's not. It's about taking care of yourself. Nowadays I only really do the things I want to do and wear the things I want to wear. Your clothes say so much about you, after all. The great thing about getting older is you don't have to do/wear/say anything you don't want to. It wasn't until my very late thirties that I stopped worrying about what other people thought. If there's one thing I've loved about getting older, it's the liberating feeling of caring less what people think about me.

From as far back as I can remember, I was always insecure about my looks. Whether it was my flat chest, my skinny legs or how to cope with my body as it changed, I never, ever loved what I looked like. Now, with the benefit of hindsight, I can see I was different. I was given a body that worked for photographic modelling and a photogenic face. Ironically, if I'd had a fairy godmother when I was fourteen, I would have begged her to make me more voluptuous and shapely. I desperately wanted bosoms, a waist, hips and to wear high-heeled pointy shoes and big skirts.

I never thought I was beautiful. I was just this funny duck-like creature with skinny legs, a face with big eyes and a blonde crop of hair on the top

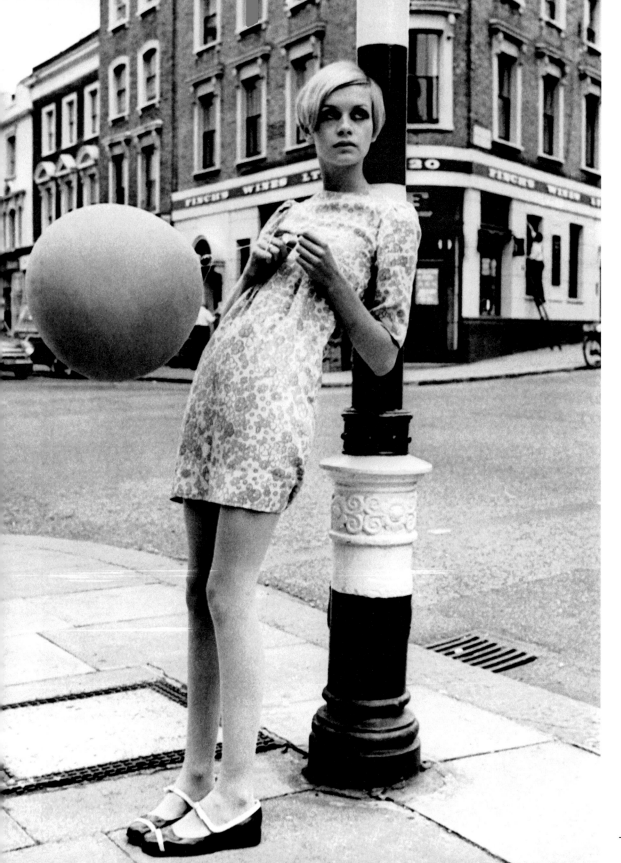

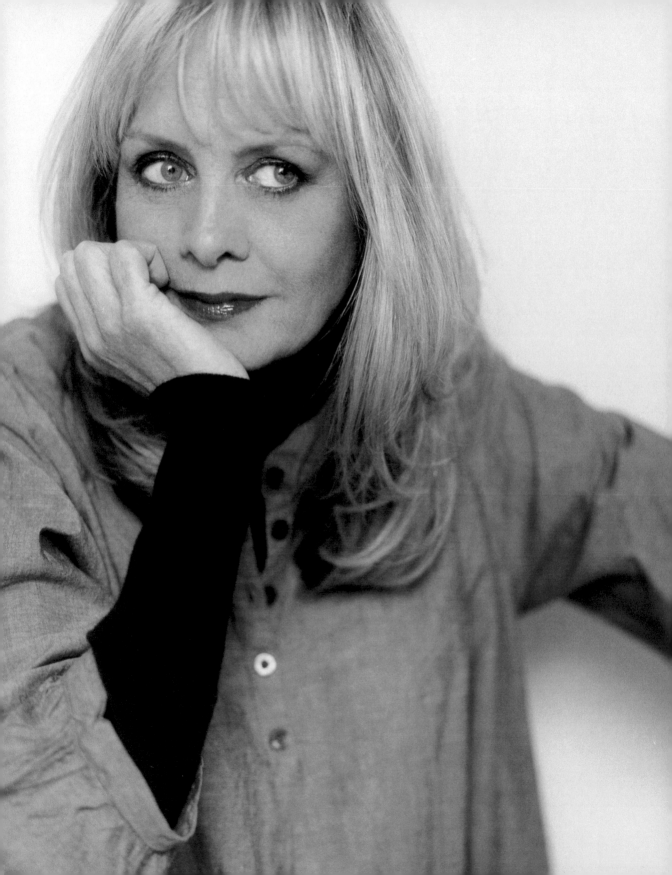

Ageing doesn't mean waving goodbye to style and individuality

Now that I really am a grown-up, what I have learned through my own experience is that every woman has something special and unique she can bring out and enhance. Look at everyone walking towards you along a street and they are all different. There's only one of them and there's only one of you. Just because you are now a grown-up woman doesn't mean you cannot look and feel beautiful, individual and different. None of these things are exclusively the domain of the very young and fresh-faced. I still don't get why everyone is so obsessed with youth and skinniness. Us older women should be able to celebrate what we wear and how we look, without feeling pressurized into fitting into a certain type.

Compared to the early years, during the time I was working my socks off, being hailed as the face of '66, when I look in the mirror now it's obviously an older face looking back at me. How I feel differs by the day. Sometimes it's 'Hmm, not so bad,' and others it's 'Oh my God, stop looking!' It doesn't matter what age you are, if you're not feeling great, you can feel like you look dreadful. Chances are, if you've had a late night and too much wine, you'll feel even worse. As us girls already know, emotions and moods directly affect the way we look. I feel the same about putting clothes on. Some days I can put together an outfit and think it's great. A couple of days later I put the same thing on and wonder what on earth I was thinking.

I started taking an interest in my own style at a young age. Ever since I was a teenager, I have made my own clothes. By the age of eleven I was learning to sew under the tuition of my mum and my two big sisters. I had started

introduction

13

off wanting to make clothes for my dolls, then by the time I was thirteen I was totally into the mod look. It was virtually impossible to buy mod clothes, so the answer was to make them myself. The first thing I made was a camel-hair coat. I was so proud of it. The mod look was very specific. It changed almost weekly. I used to go to a club above a Burton's tailoring shop in Harrow once a week. Bands like the Yardbirds, Eric Burdon and the Animals and Georgie Fame would perform, but I was more interested in seeing what the older girls on the dance floor were wearing. I'd check out their looks down to the button and copy them by making my own versions. An obsession with and love of great clothes and make-up began for me back then.

From the very first time I was booked to model for teen magazines and my early years working for American *Vogue*, right through to the campaigns and cover shoots I am involved in today, fashion has taught me that it does have magnificent powers to make any woman feel and look great. You don't need pots of money to look good and you don't have to be physically perfect in order to enjoy all the benefits of a great wardrobe. Successful dressing is mostly about attitude, loving yourself and having confidence in what you wear, knowing that it's working for your body.

This book will, hopefully, be a reference and change things around on how you go about looking good, feeling good and dressing with style — whatever your style

From the ramblings in this book you'll learn that, just like the rest of the female population, yes I'm insecure, yes I have bad days, yes I crave chocolate, yes I love a glass of wine and yes I know I should exercise more. Nobody's perfect! That's what makes each one of us so much more interesting. I'd much rather that than a sea of bland, Botoxed, physically taut and toned robots we are in danger of becoming if we try too hard to be perfect.

Fashion should be fun and not scary. For us grown-ups, it should be a time for feeling fabulous about ourselves. I am not going to pretend I am the oracle on all things. What I can do is share with you some of the things I've learned over the years about clothes, make-up, looking after myself, attitude and, most important of all, shopping!

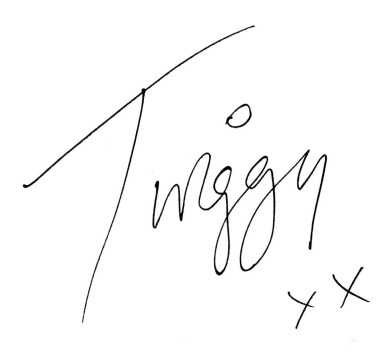

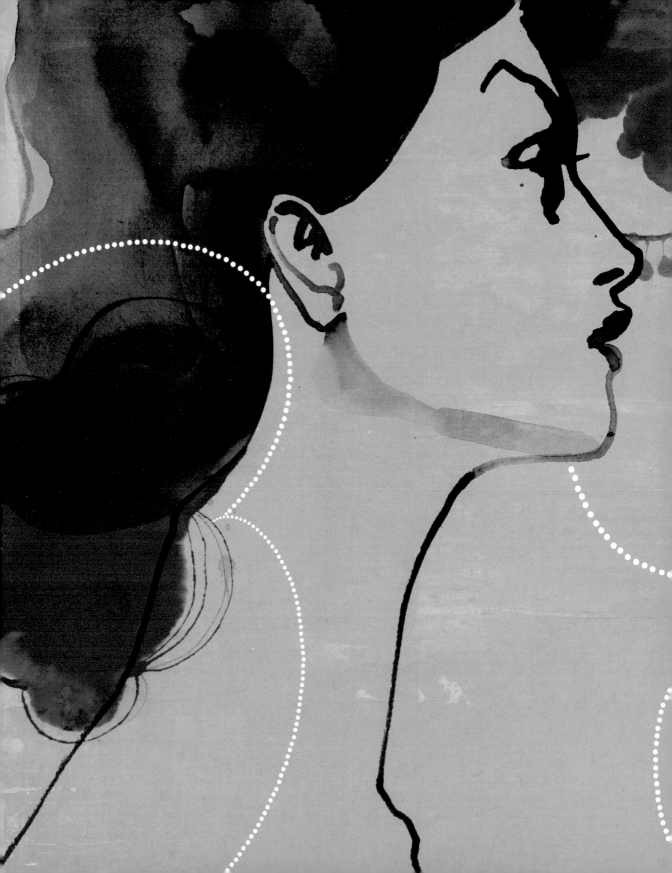

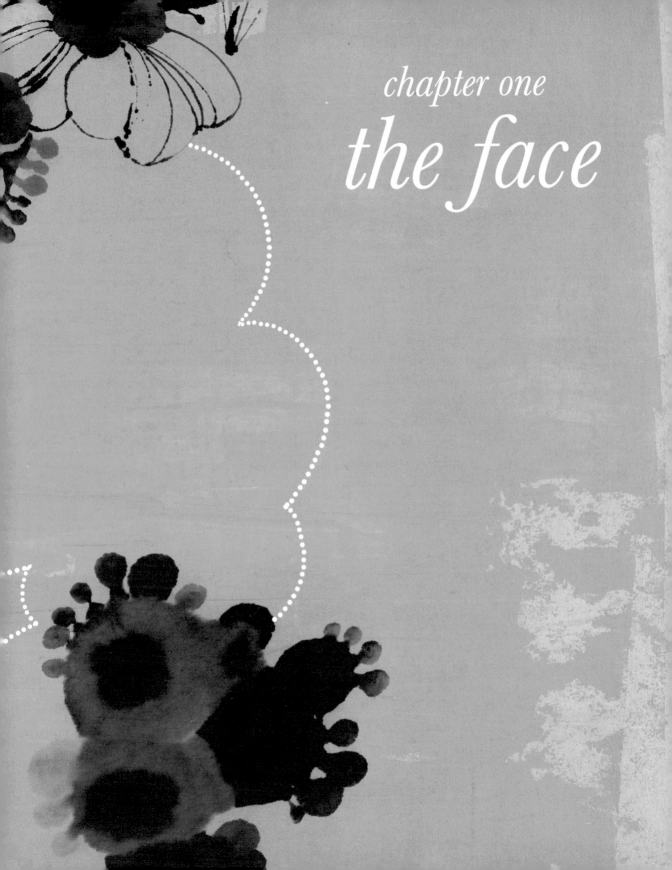

the face

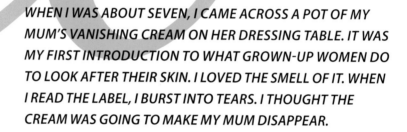

W

WHEN I WAS ABOUT SEVEN, I CAME ACROSS A POT OF MY MUM'S VANISHING CREAM ON HER DRESSING TABLE. IT WAS MY FIRST INTRODUCTION TO WHAT GROWN-UP WOMEN DO TO LOOK AFTER THEIR SKIN. I LOVED THE SMELL OF IT. WHEN I READ THE LABEL, I BURST INTO TEARS. I THOUGHT THE CREAM WAS GOING TO MAKE MY MUM DISAPPEAR.

I'm not going to say I'm in love with my wrinkles, but I've certainly learned to live with them. There's nothing wrong with them; they're a natural, inevitable part of what it means to be a human being so there's no point wishing them away. You're better off just getting on with them. To chase youth is like chasing the pot of gold at the end of the rainbow. You're never really going to find it. Follow the route of lip plumping, bum tucks, tum tucks, boob implants and Botox, and the chances are you might well end up looking like an android. Having said that, there are people who have had very subtle work done and look great. There's no doubt it does give their confidence a boost. If you are hell bent on having some cosmetic surgery, do your research, find the best surgeons,

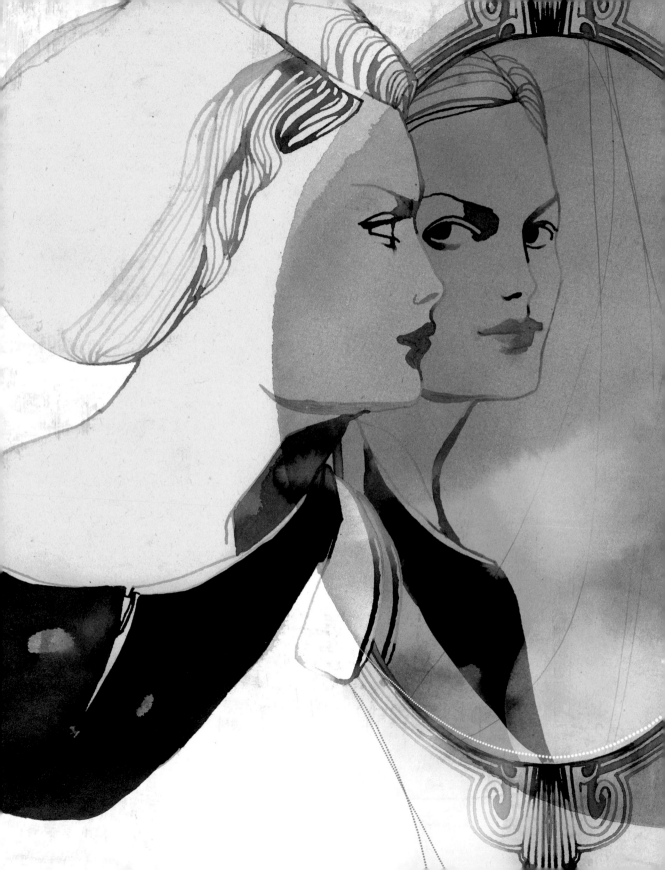

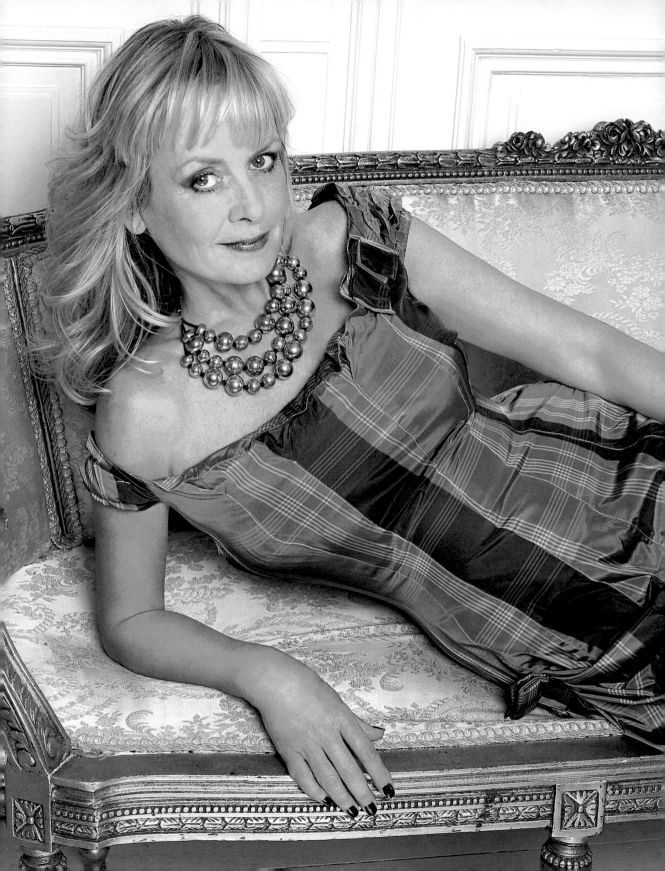

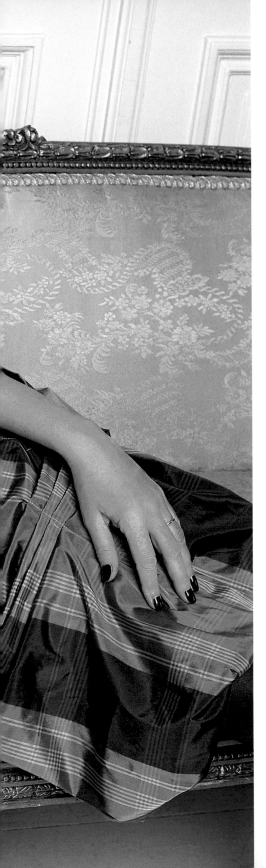

ask questions and go for subtle changes. It's also worth checking out the non-invasive procedures, which are growing daily. In the end it's a very personal choice (see p. 76 for more on this subject).

It would be foolish and naive of me to ignore the fact that we are living in a lookist, youth-oriented society, or deny that we all, including myself, love being told we look younger. At the moment, as I approach my sixtieth year on the planet, I haven't had any 'work' done, but who knows? I might get to sixty-five and have a change of heart.

Either way, women should not feel pressured into pricey cosmetic procedures to fight the inevitable, especially when so often it can require major surgery and general anaesthetic. You might argue that we're not growing old gracefully precisely because of the rise in cosmetic surgery. Everywhere we turn, the current beauty ideal is to be skinny and young. The perfection of beauty presented in advertising has been achieved with brilliant lighting, fantastic photography, make-up artists, stylists, all there to create the perfect picture. Advertising is aspirational. It's selling a dream. It's not meant to be a reality. The problem is such perfection can affect our self-esteem. It is a fact. Just remember, when you're glimpsing a billboard image of a gorgeous girl who is six feet tall and has perfect skin/ hair/eyes/figure, how this is a wonderful fantasy world meant to inspire rather than play on your insecurities.

the face

21

Just remember, when you're flicking through a magazine, how each one of these images represents a wonderful fantasy world

Despite knowing this, even the most intelligent woman can look at herself in the mirror and decide that anything veering from 'perfect' is a failure. And it often feels that the older we get, the harder it is to achieve the perfection. But it's not, nor should it be! Apparently, the ancient Egyptians had the odd nose job, so plastic surgery is obviously not new. There is nothing modern about the desire to transform and improve ourselves. What is new – and is something I believe to be a welcome development – is the increased sophistication in non-invasive procedures that no longer require incisions, cuts, bruises and scars. It is how you feel about your looks that is the key to happiness and a healthy self-esteem.

Every wrinkle tells a story. Among them are the laughter lines, which crinkle when a woman smiles, and those are wonderful. They add character and depth to a woman's face. In my opinion, there's nothing worse than a blank, overly Botoxed face with no expression. Some young people look absolutely awful, whereas some older women look drop-dead gorgeous! It's all a state of mind. However, the skin does need looking after and tending to. It is the largest organ in the body, after all.

By the time we reach our forties, it's hard to change the habits of a lifetime. I've got the driest skin on the planet and as a result have used quite a rich face cream ever since I was a teenager. I'm emotionally attached to my moisturizer. It's an old friend. It's not

For this vital chapter, I consulted my great friend, the cosmetic designer and make-up artist Barbara Daly

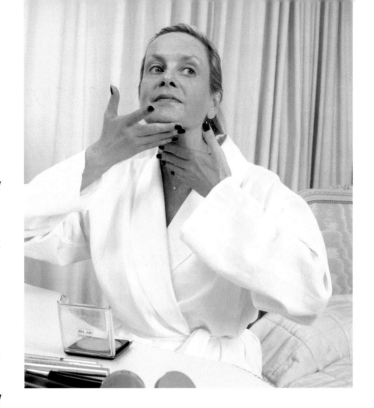

necessarily the best or most expensive one in the world, but it works for me. There are so many fabulous creams out there and some of the great ones don't cost the earth.

BARBARA DALY, make-up artists MARY GREENWELL and KAY MONTANO, and a number of dermatologists provided me with some invaluable tips on skincare:

'The ageing process can bring all sorts of changes to the skin,' says Kay Montano. 'On the face, the skin tends to get thinner and finer. It loses elasticity and overall it does not reflect light any more. Young skin has more moisture in it than older skin. As we age, the epidermis loses its plumpness and the outer layer of skin gets finer. Nearly all anti-ageing creams try to plump the outer layer of the skin.'

the face

LIGHT REFLECTORS
YOU MIGHT LIKE TO TRY

LUXURY
- *Armani Fluid Sheer*
- *Prescriptives Magic Illuminating Liquid Potion*

MIDDLE
- *Clinique Up-lighting Liquid Illuminator*

BUDGET
- *Revlon Skinlights*
- *Barbara Daly for Tesco Soft-focus Light Reflecting Base*

We should all know by now that drinking water is one of the best things we can do for our skin. I find drinking water such a chore. Sleeping with heating on can add three years to your face, simply due to your skin being dried to a crisp overnight. Fresh air helps you sleep better too, but if it's a necessity to have those radiators pumping, put a humidifier in the room or place a bowl of water on the radiator to replenish the dry air with moisture.

It is not just how we keep our skin hydrated that matters, but also how we use the right products to give it a healthy glow. If you are the same age as me, the way you wear make-up is likely to have been set in stone a long time ago. In which case, it could be time for an update.

'Fashions change but so does the skin,' says Kay. 'Heavy Natural' was a big trend ten to fifteen years ago. Remember when taupe, beige and brown shades were all the rage? Cut to ten years later when our skin is becoming more matt and dull, and many women who were in their thirties at the peak of that trend are still using overly matt taupes/terracotta bronzes/peaches that absorb light and don't bounce off the skin.'

One of the biggest steps forward in cosmetics in recent years is the development of products with light-reflecting particles. These are not to be confused with shimmer and shine products.

Kay says, 'With make-up there are all kinds of tools that help to create an optical illusion. Women often think make-up is about what colour you use, what trends are hot and how to apply those to your face. But the real skill of make-up is the stuff that's less obvious, such as making your skin look really amazing and luminous, and concealing blemishes and pigmentation issues without looking like you've got make-up on.'

According to Mary Greenwell, the main crime us girls make as we get older is ignoring the importance of wearing the right foundation.

'It's trial and error to find the right one, but it should blend easily and become part of your skin, not a mask. You'll instantly look more glowing and youthful.'

'Covering your skin with heavy foundation is the most ageing thing you can do,' says Barbara Daly. 'Often you don't need to wear foundation all over, just around the nose and on the chin. And put concealer on afterwards, or you'll wipe it all away.'

'The best tip about anti-ageing make-up is to use your products to make yourself look healthy. Do this and you instantly look younger'
KAY MONTANO

eyes

I'VE ALWAYS DONE MY OWN EYE MAKE-UP. THE FIRST TIME I EVER PICKED UP A MASCARA BRUSH WAS BACK IN MY MOD PHASE WHEN I WAS FOURTEEN. It was a very specific look, heavy round the eyes. This was only at weekends as wearing make-up at school was strictly verboten. I'd meet up with my friends and mess about with eyeblack – a pot of solid black liner mixed with a bit of spit on the end of a fine brush.

A lot of mainstream eyeshadows back then were pale green, pale blue and soft beige. I wanted smokey eyes like the screen goddesses from the 1930s, so I scoured the shops for dark shades. Thank goodness BIBA make-up came out about that time, with all the smokey shades of chocolate-brown, grey and more black.

I still use those colours today. The difference is that back then I was layering three pairs of false eyelashes over my own. Underneath the lashes, I'd paint extra 'twigs' onto my skin with the eyeblack. I got the idea for them from my school friend's rag doll. The whole process used to take me an hour and a half. I'd start with a very fine black line in the top of the eye socket, following the shape of the bone. I would let it dry, and blend in the eye-shadow above it. On the top lid, I would draw another very fine black line near my own lashes, coming out to the corner and joining the top bit, leaving the lid completely pale. Then I would apply the false lashes. The final touch was blocking out my lips with pancake, a hangover from the mod days. When I started modelling, on the days I was working I would set the alarm for ninety minutes before I had to leave the front door, as it took that long to apply the make-up. I loved every minute of it. It was so therapeutic and such fun.

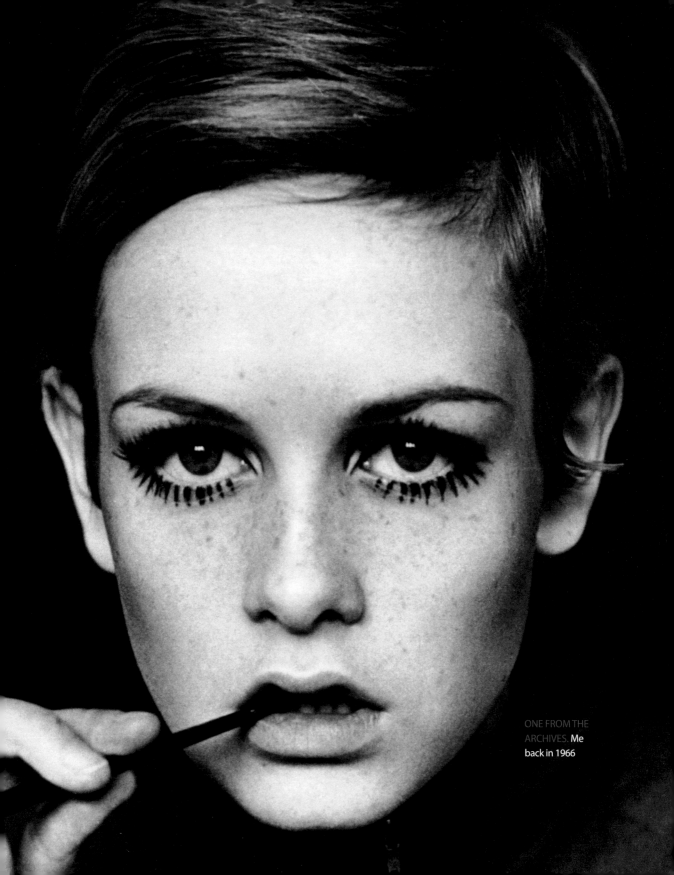

ONE FROM THE
ARCHIVES. Me
back in 1966

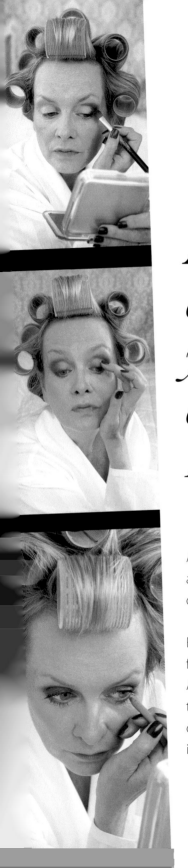

A little bit of make-up is always going to enhance your features. I wear quite a lot of eye make-up when I go out and it works for me

A lot of older women I have met think that once they're past a certain age they shouldn't be too made up. I agree when it comes to foundation, and we'll cover that later.

For some women, the idea of wearing make-up fills them with fear, but it's a good way to draw attention to your best features. At the very least, mascara can open up the eyes and add depth to your face. As you get older, not wearing any make-up at all can leave you looking tired. But how you do your own make-up is such a personal thing.

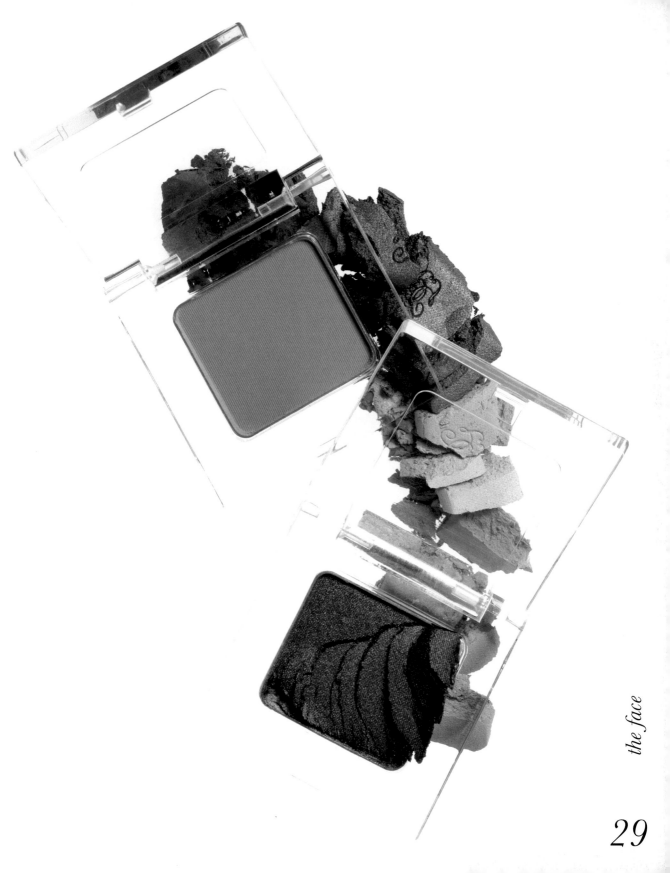

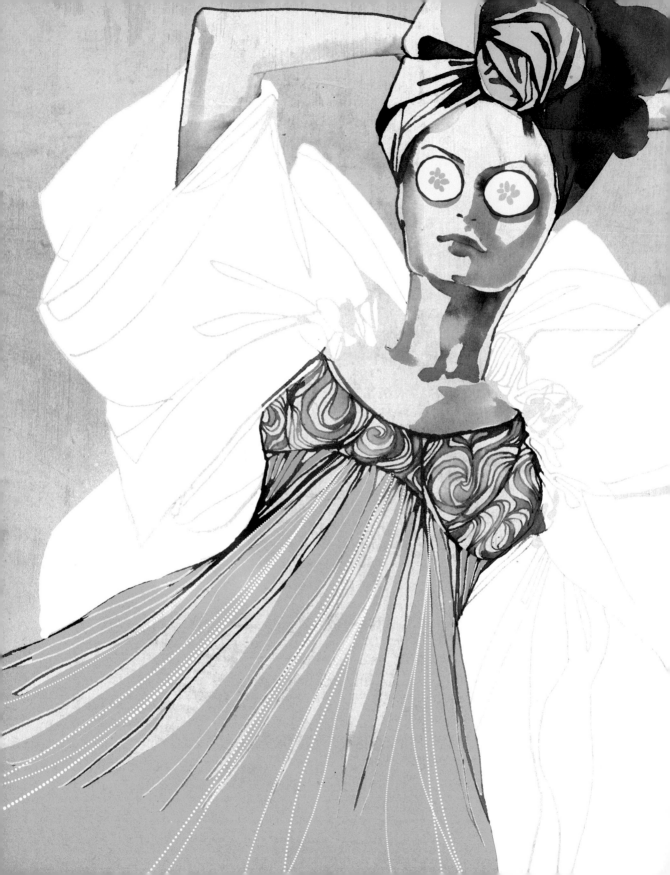

UNDER EYE & CIRCLES

ACCORDING TO OUR EXPERT TEAM, WHEN YOU'RE YOUNGER, YOU CAN PRETTY MUCH USE ANY COVER-UP. As you age, skin under the eyes gets superfine so dry cover-up no longer works as a texture. In fact, it will accentuate wrinkles. Luckily, a whole new style of under-eye concealers – **YSL'S TOUCHE ÉCLAT RADIANT TOUCH CONCEALER** was the first – in finer, more liquid formulations are available and suit skin of any age. I always stock up on **TOUCHE ÉCLAT** at the airport. It's one of my make-up staples. When we are younger, dark circles can look cute and mysterious, but you can't get away with it post-forty. It just makes you look old and tired! *(See our section on Concealers, p. 54.)*

BRIGHT EYES

IN OUR AGE GROUP WE ALL WORRY ABOUT OUR FACE DROPPING A LITTLE BIT. Gravity is a fact of living on the planet. It's what keeps our feet on the ground and, as we age, certain other parts of the body can start to droop downwards. I always say it takes me a few hours for my face to get out of its sleep shape and into its daytime shape. One of the things that I find a challenge from time to time is puffy eyes. When I wake up before my eyes do, I grab a bag of frozen peas from the freezer and alternate holding it over each eye. I can often be eating my toast at breakfast with one eye under the peas. If I'm travelling and have been stuck in a hotel without the frozen peas, a couple of small cans from the minibar fridge rolled gently over the eye sockets works wonders. Just hope nobody rings your door! Cucumber slices and refrigerated, squeezed-out tea bags also work wonders on puffy eyes.

If you feel the need to use oil-based eye creams, don't slather your eyelids in the product as it can make them swell. According to Kay, a good rule is not to apply eye creams any closer to the eye than the bone. Pat the cream very gently around the bone area, circling the whole eye. The skin is so delicate it will be absorbed.

the face

EYE CREAMS
YOU MIGHT
LIKE TO TRY

LUXURY
- *La Prairie Cellular Radiance Eye Cream*

MIDDLE
- *Roc Retin-Ox+ Eye Intensive Anti-wrinkle Cream*
- *Prescriptives Vibrant-C Brightening Eye Cream*

BUDGET
- *L'Oréal Paris Revitalift Double Lifting Eye*
- *Olay Regenerist Eye Lifting Serum*

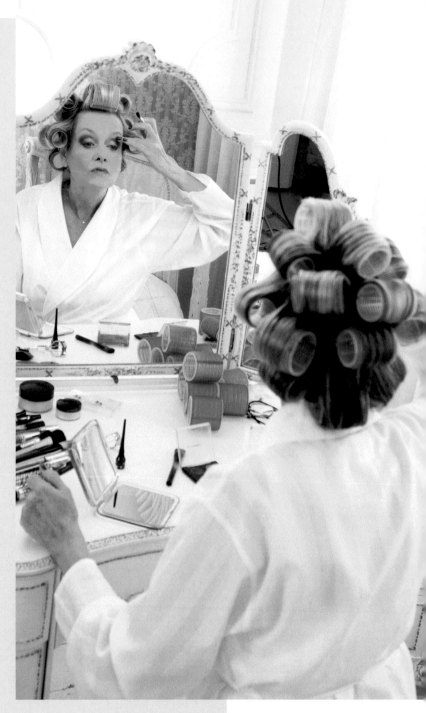

MASCARA & EYELASHES

EYELASHES ARE OFTEN FORGOTTEN ABOUT BY THE OLDER GENERATION but they play a vital role in drawing the attention to the face.

'Even if your eyes are quite hooded, a bit of mascara perks them up,' says Kay. 'Perkiness is something you lose as you age. The desire to look perky and vibrant then becomes a mission.'

With this in mind, invest in an eyelash curler. It's our number-one experts' tip for perking up the face. As you get older, you want to try anything to create upwards movement on the face. Another suggestion is to use clear mascara on the eyebrows and brush them upwards. I agree about the eyelash curlers and my added tip is to gently heat them with a hair dryer. But please test on your hand and make sure it's not burning your skin before applying to the eyelash. Better still, invest in the heated eyelash curlers available. It's amazing how much they curl with that little bit of heat.

'Heated eyelash curlers are great, but the first thing to do is learn to use eyelash curlers properly,' says Barbara. 'Make sure you've got the good ones with a nice pad so you don't crack the lashes. You want to get them as close to the roots as possible so you don't bend the ends into an L shape. The big trick when you squeeze the curlers together is don't be nervous about pressing quite hard. Once you have pressed them and done the "curl", open the curlers back up properly before you remove them – you don't want to drag half of your eyelashes off with them. Don't panic if there's the odd lash on the curler as they do renew every five or six weeks. As you get older, lashes get shorter, so curling not only brightens eyes and opens them up, it's very youthful as it makes lashes look longer. You can either put one coat of mascara on before you curl, to make it hold for longer, or apply afterwards.'

MASCARAS
YOU MIGHT LIKE TO TRY

HIGH
- *Lancôme still does the best, from Hypnôse to L'Extrême and Amplicils – pick the one that's right for your eyelashes*

MIDDLE
- *Clinique High Impact Mascara*
- *Estée Lauder Projectionist High Definition Volume Mascara*

BUDGET
- *Max Factor Masterpiece Mascara*
- *Maybelline Volum' Express*

The **SHU UEMURA EYELASH CURLER** is the one every make-up artist swears by; the silicone pads make sure your lashes are protected. Boots have a great selection of heated eyelash curlers, including their own **NO. 7**, or try eye-care experts **TALIKA'S HEATED EYELASH CURLER**.

False eyelashes are fabulous for evening wear but can be tricky to apply. Be very careful not to get glue in your eye. The individual lashes are easier to put on. If, like most of my girlfriends, you would rather leave it to the professionals, you can always go to your nearest salon early evening and have them applied by an expert. It won't take long and, if you've got a really special occasion, it's well worth the extra effort of getting them done for you. It doesn't cost much and transforms your eyes in a spectacular way. Look for volumizing, thickening mascaras to give lashes back their fullness.

Tinting your eyelashes at a salon is also worth considering for a low maintenance, high impact treat. It means you don't always have to apply mascara and it makes such a difference. It's a great thing to do before you go on holiday, so you don't have to keep applying mascara and you can swim at will.

The minute you use eyelash curlers, it lifts and opens the eyes

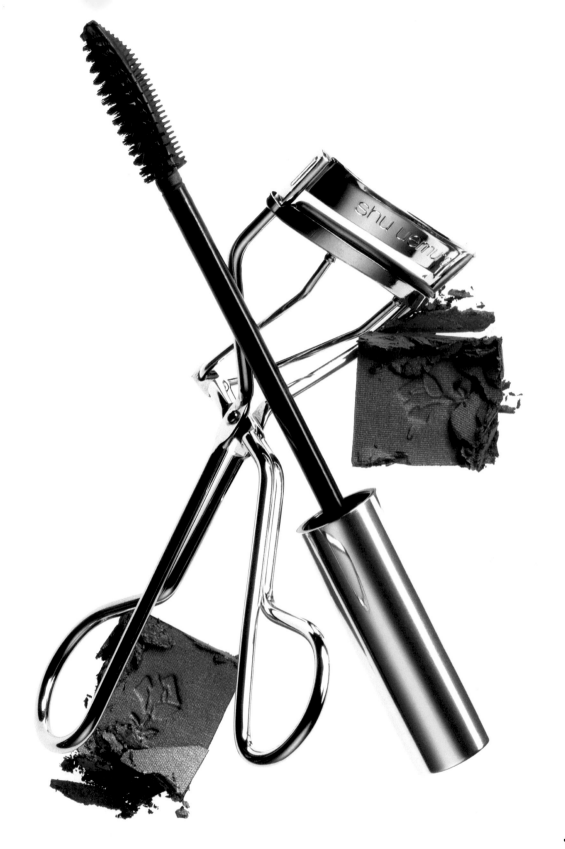

I CAN SEE
CLEARLY NOW

UNTIL I WAS ABOUT FORTY-FIVE MY VISION WAS FINE.
Then I started needing glasses to read. If you have this
problem, the other great thing to invest in is a
magnified make-up mirror. I've used one for many years
and it's fantastic. They come in various strengths, 3x , 5x,
7x and so on. Find the one that suits your eyes. They are
available from John Lewis and all good chemists and
department stores.

*Your brows
should help
form an
arch to the
bridge of
the nose*

EYEBROWS

IN 1970 I WAS CAST TO STAR IN MY FIRST FILM, *THE
BOYFRIEND*, DIRECTED BY KEN RUSSELL. The film was
set in the 1920s. For the movie I plucked my eyebrows
quite drastically in order to create the 1920s look. The
outer edges never grew back. I'm not a hairy person and
have always plucked the odd stray ones. If you do have
uneven or stray eyebrows but are not brave enough
to attempt plucking them yourself, threading is a great
alternative. This is an Indian technique whereby hairs are
literally pulled out using cotton threads. It is said to be less
ageing in the long term, as it pulls the skin much less than
tweezing does.

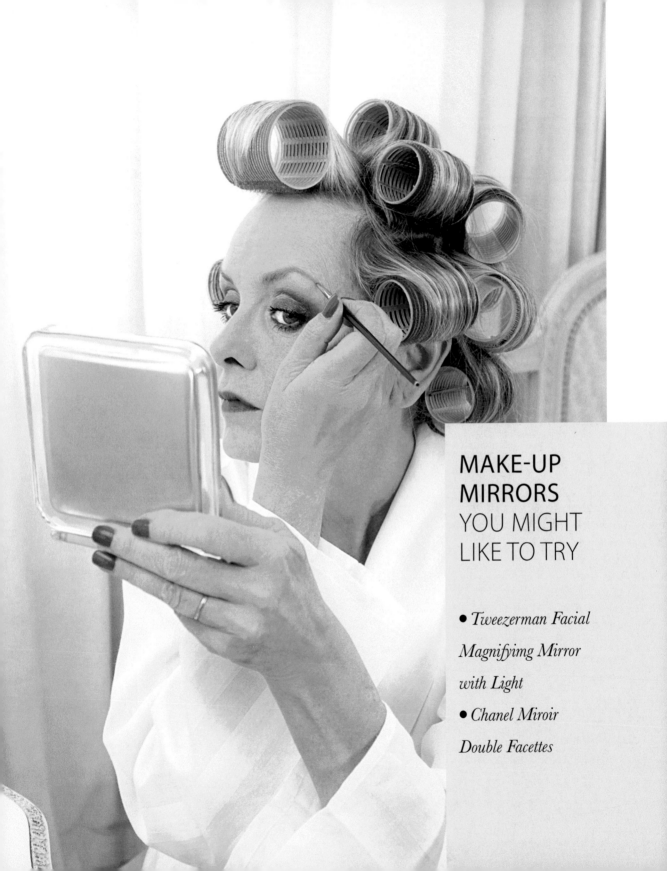

MAKE-UP
MIRRORS
YOU MIGHT
LIKE TO TRY

- *Tweezerman Facial Magnifyimg Mirror with Light*
- *Chanel Miroir Double Facettes*

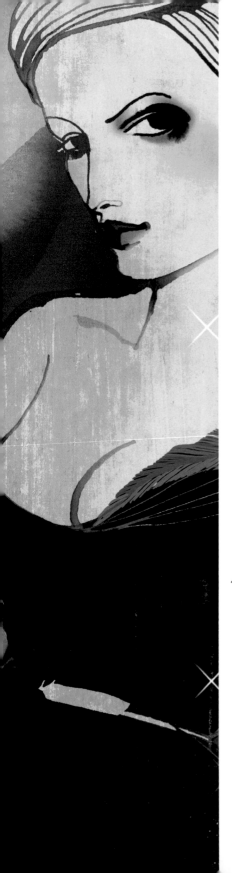

Lots of us make the mistake of plucking our eyebrows too far apart.

'Don't!' says Barbara. 'It instantly makes your eyes look smaller. The apostrophe shape is very unnatural and makes you look surprised and a bit angry! If you do pluck them at home, look at both eyebrows at the same time, do a bit of one, then the other. The line underneath shouldn't be too thin. For novices I'd always advise to see a professional. Once we reach our forties, the muscle in the brow can start to slacken. Shaping the brows properly can be the perfect way to give them an instant lift.'

Unless you have naturally dark, heavy eyebrows, a soft, gentle pencilling-in is better than a heavy line.

Here are Barbara Daly's brow tips:

1 **MOST PEOPLE'S BROW COLOUR DIFFERS FROM THEIR HAIR COLOUR,** so don't buy brow pencils to match your hair, pick a product that matches your brow colour.

2 **IF YOUR BROWS ARE GOING GREY,** choose a soft colour to cover, such as BOBBI BROWN'S NATURAL BROW SHAPER, to brush on colour. Better still, have them tinted.

THREADING

THE KEY TO GETTING THE EYEBROWS YOU WANT IS COMMUNICATION WITH YOUR BEAUTICIAN. Tell them how you like your brows to be, whether it's thick and full, natural, groomed, etc. Tell them what you're scared of: too thin, too far apart, too arched.

Threading is an ancient technique of hair removal that came over from India. One of the pioneers of threading in the UK is **KAMINI**, whose salon is off Kensington Church Street in London. Kamini is passionate about the benefits of threading and her eventual aim is that her clients will only have to come to see her every six months to a year, as she 'trains' the stray hairs in their brows not to grow back. The whole process takes about fifteen minutes, with Kamini whisking away hairs with two threads. Her only demand is that you don't pluck in between, as you'll interfere with her master plan for your brows. She's a perfectionist who believes less is more. She is the person to see to get a natural shape.

VAISHALY is London's other favourite threader (and facialist). She creates a polished eyebrow, perfect for women who like to appear well groomed. For regional threading contact your local spa.

PLUCKING, WAXING, TATTOOING

THERE IS NOTHING WRONG WITH WAXING YOUR BROWS. Some people claim it pulls the skin more than plucking, but it gives lovely results. Sophie Thorpe is a shaping, waxing and semi-permanent make-up expert, who will correct brows that have been over-plucked, made uneven by scars or affected by medication. 'The difference getting your brows back can make to your face is remarkable,' says Sophie. 'It opens the eyes right up, gives you structure and means you have to wear less make-up to look pulled together.' If you've really overdone the plucking, or suffered hair loss from alopecia or chemotherapy, you may have heard of eyebrow tattooing. This is semi-permanent and sounds terrifying but the experts rave about Sophie. She painstakingly fills in individual hairs and the results look natural and wonderful for any of us who simply have no brow hair at all.

the face

39

skin tones

<u>THIS IS KAY'S TIP:</u> *TAKE A GOOD LOOK AT YOUR FACE IN NATURAL DAYLIGHT. DO YOU HAVE ANY BROKEN VEINS? IS YOUR SKIN HIGHLY PIGMENTED? IF SO, MAKE AN APPOINTMENT TO SEE A DERMATOLOGIST FOR ADVICE AND RELEVANT TREATMENT.*

Try to be honest with yourself. The way you use make-up may well benefit from an update, not least because the face changes shape as we get older. Where you used to apply blusher may not be appropriate any more. Take a good look at how your skin has changed and note the areas you feel might need a little help.

Whatever you do, don't rely on a department store makeover where the emphasis can be on selling you the product and not on providing you with what's best for you. Make-up companies tend to operate on a one-size-fits-all basis, so you might end up with a product that's not right. A common mistake is to confuse dehydrated skin with dry skin. Women who do this will use richer creams that make them spotty when in fact they need a hydrating moisturizer.

INSTEAD, ASK YOURSELF THE FOLLOWING THREE QUESTIONS:

the face

1. What would you like improved?

2. Do you have uneven skin colour?

3. Is it dry, oily, combination, sensitive?

Once you have established your skin type, you can set about a routine that will help to look after it and keep it glowing and healthy.

One of the best things you could also do is to visit a make-up expert for non-biased tips on how to make the most of your features.

MAKE-UP EXPERTS YOU MIGHT LIKE TO TRY

● **KAY MONTANO**
provides excellent private masterclasses and group workshops.

● **MARY GREENWELL**
is now giving classes to teach women all her brilliant tricks and helps you create both a day and an evening look.

● **JEMMA KIDD**
has started her own wonderful make-up school where she runs non-professional make-up masterclasses, including the 'fabulous at forty and beyond'.

CLEANSING

I LOVE THIS PART OF MY DAILY ROUTINE. Cleansing the skin is the best thing you can do, morning and night. It helps to remove dead cells, is a way to gently exfoliate and to unwind. Try to breathe deeply while you cleanse, as bringing extra oxygen to the body is relaxing and good for you. If you cleansed well the night before, a hot flannel pressed to the face with a few deep breaths is just as good a way to wake up the skin as any. Remember to include your neck in this daily routine! Drier than your face, your neck needs as much love and care, if not more, to help stave off sagging and drooping. Finish off with a cool flannel compress. If you are using a lotion, enjoy the feeling of your chosen cleanser circulating over the face and neck. Never scrub or rub hard and always apply it in upward strokes/circles to help fight gravity.

When I cleanse at night, I use a rich moisturizer to remove make-up with a tissue. Once I have done that, I apply more moisturizer as my skin is so dry. In the mornings, I always like to splash my face with cold water to wake me up. It helps refresh me and also helps with that still-asleep feeling around the eyes. I pat my face dry, then immediately slather on the moisturizer.

Massaging your skin helps with circulation, which can bring a bit of bloom to the face

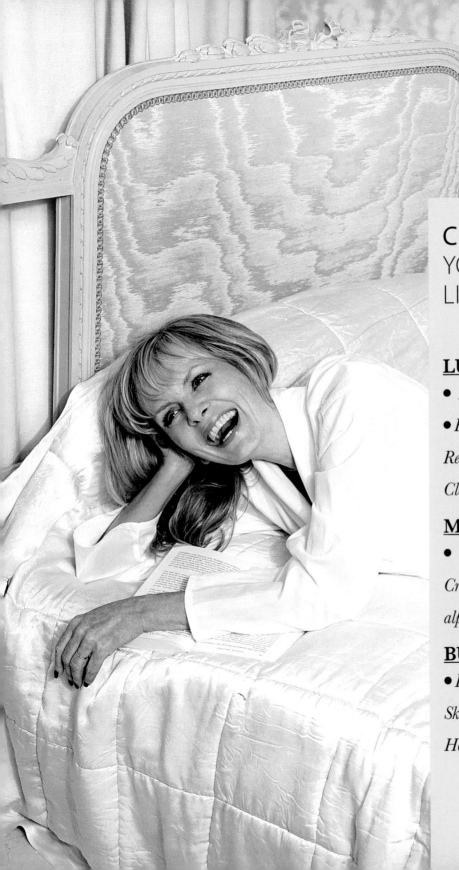

CLEANSERS
YOU MIGHT
LIKE TO TRY

LUXURY
- *Eve Lom Cleanser*
- *Prescriptives Intensive Rebuilding Moisture Rich Cleanser*

MIDDLE
- *Skinceuticals Cleansing Cream (with skin-sloughing alpha hydroxy acids)*

BUDGET
- *Liz Earle Naturally Active Skincare Cleanse and Polish Hot Cloth Cleanser*

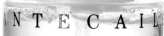

WELEDA

WILD
ROS

gently purifies
and invigorates

Lotion tonique
pour le visage

purifie et
vivifie délicatement

For intensive nourishment
Soin nourissant intensif

100 ml ℮ 3.4 FL OZ

Eau de
Rose de Mai

Pure Rosewater

Jurlique

Rosewater
Balancing
Mist

℮ 100mL 3.3 fl.oz.

TONING

HAVING VERY DRY SKIN, I HAVE NEVER USED A TONER.
Beauty experts warn that many toners simply strip the skin of its natural oils and are best avoided. My alternative to a toner is a flannel compress, using the same cleansing cloth as mentioned after cleansing but rinsed in cool water instead of hot. If you do like toners, go for gentle, alcohol-free products such as **LIZ EARLE**, **DR HAUSCHKA** and **CHANTECAILLE**.

MOISTURIZING

MY SKIN HAS ALWAYS BEEN VERY DRY SO I'M FOREVER SLAPPING ON THE MOISTURIZER. I can't bear the feeling of a taut, dry face. According to Dr David Colbert, New York-based dermatologist to Oscar-winning movie stars and Brit supermodels, nothing dries the skin faster than menopause. Now is the time to bump up your moisturizer. Look out for products containing shea butter or lecithin, a natural fat, which dissolves effortlessly and feeds parched skin.

As our skin becomes drier with age it is so important to regularly moisturize the neck and décolletage. There are many creams specifically targeted to this delicate area of skin.

TONERS YOU MIGHT LIKE TO TRY

LUXURY
- *Chantecaille Pure Rosewater*

MIDDLE
- *Caudalie Eau de Beauté*
- *Jurlique Rosewater*

BUDGET
- *Weleda Iris or Wild Rose Facial Toner*

MOISTURIZERS
YOU MIGHT LIKE TO TRY

1 *Dry to Normal*

LUXURY

- *Crème de la Mer*
- *Guerlain Orchidée Impériale*
- *Estée Lauder Re-Nutriv Ultimate Lifting Crème*

MIDDLE

- *Clarins Advanced Extra Firming Day Lotion SPF 15*
- *Kiehl's Lycopene Facial Moisturizing Cream*
- *Dr Hauschka Rose Day Cream Light*
- *REN Osmotic Infusion Ultra Moisture Day Cream*

BUDGET

- *Neal's Yard Frankincense Nourishing Cream*
- *Astral Cream*

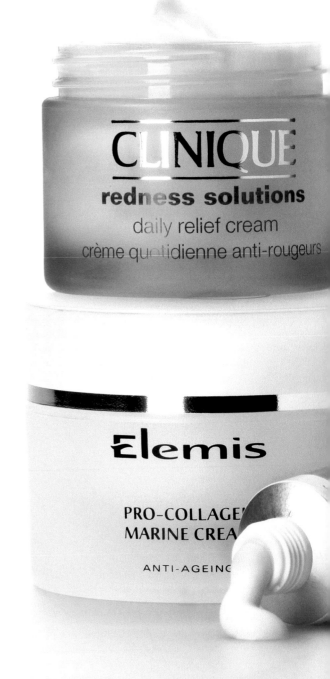

2 Oily

LUXURY

- *Leaf & Rusher Tx Acne 1.2.3 Collection*

MIDDLE

- *Dr. Brandt Poreless Moisture*
- *Dermalogica Active Moist*

BUDGET

- *Neutrogena Visibly Clear Oil-Free Moisturizer*

3 Combination

LUXURY

- *Sisley Hydra-Global Hydration Intense Anti-Age*

MIDDLE

- *Elemis Pro-collagen Marine Cream*

BUDGET

- *Nivea Visage Anti-wrinkle Q10 Plus*

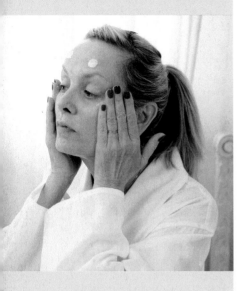

4 *Sensitive*

LUXURY

● *La Prairie Cellular Nurturing Cream Anti-redness*

MIDDLE

● *Clinique Redness Solutions Daily Relief Cream*

BUDGET

●*Aveeno Ultra-Calming Moisturizing Cream*

Make sure you have patted the skin dry before applying moisturizer. Don't rub it in like mad; instead squeeze some into the palm of your hand, lightly rub it between your hands to cover both of them, then gently press the moisturizer onto your face, starting from the décolletage and working your way upwards. Sounds a bit barmy but it really works. You may need to reapply your moisturizer to your hands in stages, first for the neck area, then the face. About twice a month I apply pure vitamin E oil after moisturizing at night. It helps keep the skin soft. You might like to try mixing a sun-screen cream into your favourite moisturizer for added protection from the elements during the daytime. Otherwise, **DERMALOGICA SOLAR DEFENSE BOOSTER SPF 30** and **BECCA'S OIL-FREE MINERAL SPF 30 MAKE-UP PRIMER** are highly recommended.

As we get older, it is so important to include the neck and décolletage whenever we moisturize

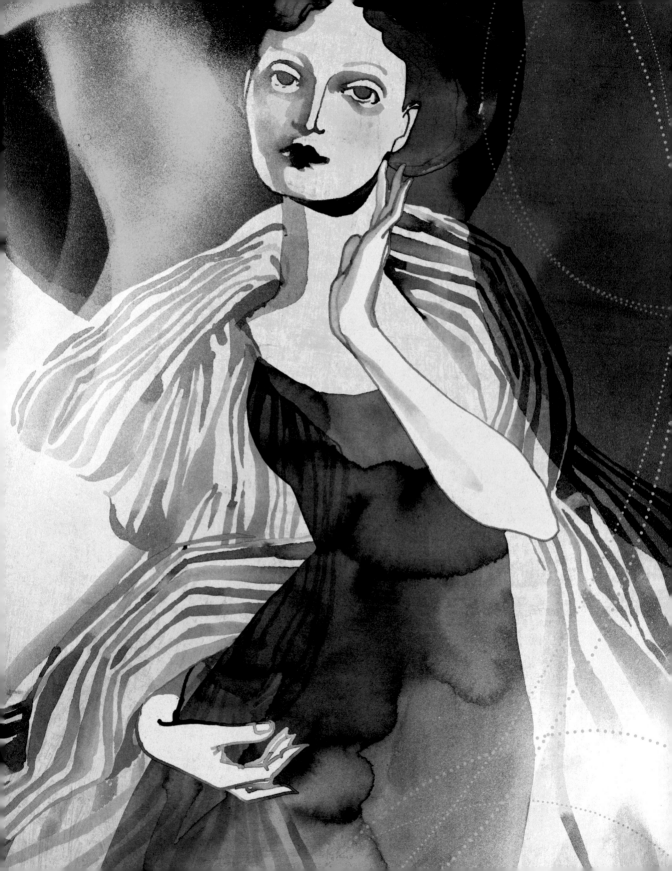

FOUNDATIONS

A LIGHT FOUNDATION CAN BE ONE OF THE OLDER WOMAN'S BEAUTY LIFE-SAVERS. The most important trick is to match the tint to your skin tone and never, ever choose a foundation in a store with artificial light. Kay suggests the following:

'Lightly dot the shades you think match your skin along the lower cheek, just above the jawline. Go outside into daylight with a mirror and pick the one that matches your skin. Never ever choose a foundation in a shop before taking this test.'

The reason for this is that most people have perfect skin in that area of the face, but the only way to truly know if your foundation shade matches it is to check it in the truthful glare of daylight.

1. Even coverage

If you are applying base, make sure the foundation is not too heavy. Keep it light. Sometimes it can be enough either to use a tinted moisturizer or to mix your favourite moisturizer with a squirt of foundation and create a lighter coverage. Always start in the middle of the face, either with your fingers or with a sponge around the nose (where we tend to go most red) and work outwards, remembering to check for 'tide marks' at the edge of the face. Blend, blend, blend. Foundation doesn't make your skin look younger, but if you use the right combination of products overall you can create the optical illusion of youthful bloom.

2. Blend-it-yourself and tinted moisturizers

An alternative to foundation can be creating your own tinted moisturizer. A friend of mine does this and creates a fabulous, light coverage. First she slathers her face in moisturizer to ensure there is no dryness. In the palm of her hand she then mixes a squirt of her favourite foundation with two squirts of a hydrating moisturizer or make-up primer, and applies this to her face with her fingertips.

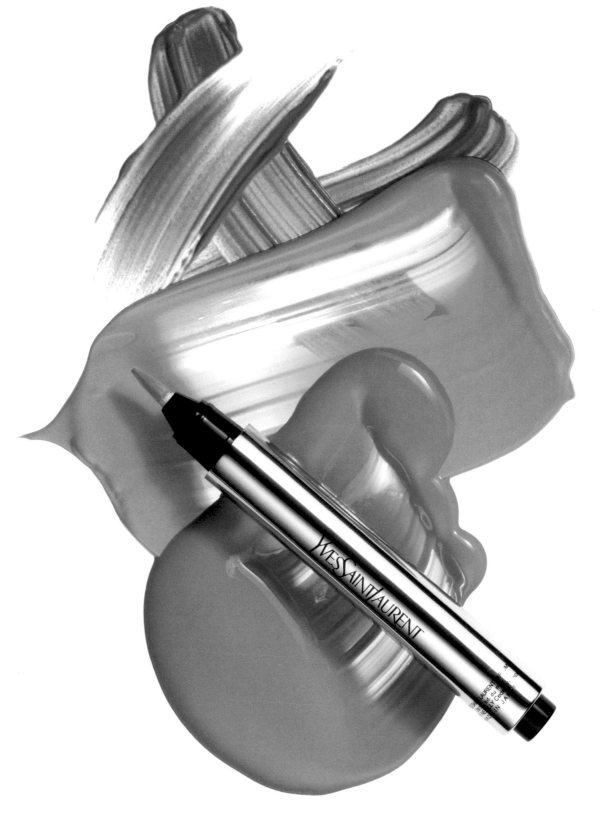

51

Even the most beautiful women in the world have relied on clever make-up tricks to enhance their looks

It used to be the case that tinted moisturizers made you look like you were using fake tan, but not now. Some of the best foundation alternatives are the latest tinted moisturizers. Beauty editor, Antonia Whyatt, mixes **PRESCRIPTIVES MAGIC ILLUMINATING LIQUID POTION** with her foundation.

'Swirl them together in the palm of your hand and apply. It will light up your face without looking too shiny,' she says.

It's easy to get bogged down by the imperfections of our skin as we age. Even film stars have been known to take painstaking measures to make themselves look younger. One such woman was Marlene Dietrich. Her technique for lifting the features was extreme. She would plait the hair tufts on either side of her face at the temples and above her ears, then pull both small plaits as tight as she could and secure them upwards, thereby lifting her face and creating a tightening of skin. As part of a well-known Hollywood trick, a wig would then have been placed on top of the pinned-back hair to complete the glamour moment. Rumour has it that the same silver-screen goddess also used a gold chain under the jawline to pull up her jowls. Due to the light being above her head at all times, this chain was never seen on screen. Do not attempt to do this at home – you might hang yourself! The reason she looked so extraordinarily perfect was that it was a grand illusion. I have heard of other movie stars who insisted on a pair of tights being fixed over the lens to ensure they stayed young and fresh-looking. Find solace in this and know that we all need a little bit of help!

FOUNDATIONS
YOU MIGHT LIKE TO TRY

LUXURY
- *Chantecaille Real Skin Foundation*

MIDDLE
- *Clinique Gentle Light Make-up*
- *Organic Pharmacy Organic Glam Luminous Antioxidant Foundation*

BUDGET
- *Bourjois 10 Hour Sleep Effect Foundation*

TINTED MOISTURIZERS
YOU MIGHT LIKE TO TRY

LUXURY
- *Laura Mercier Tinted Moisturizer SPF 20*

MIDDLE
- *Bobbi Brown Extra SPF 25 Tinted Moisturizing Balm*
- *Clarins Hydra Care Tinted Moisturizer*

BUDGET
- *Boots Botanics Instant Glow Moisturizer*

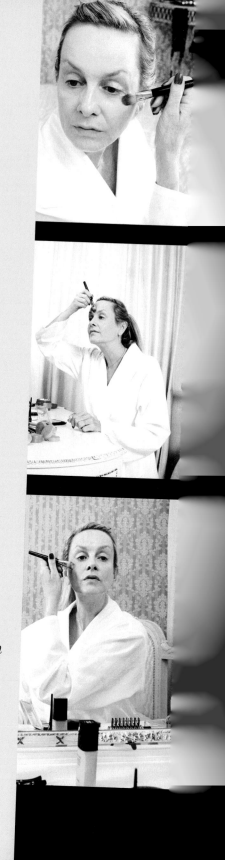

CONCEALER

'IF THERE IS ONE ESSENTIAL COSMETIC FOR OLDER SKIN, IT'S CONCEALER,' SAYS BARBARA.

And she's right. We may not have pimples, but that doesn't mean we are blemish-free and flawless. Blotches, dark patches, pigmentation – all these things benefit from a little extra attention from clever concealing tricks. The key with concealers is to match the shades to your natural skin tone.

Around the eyes most women's skin is one shade lighter than their overall skin tone. This means the foundation you use on your face may not be appropriate for around the eyes, and anyway it can be too heavy for this part of your face. Under the eyes there can often be discoloration.

'Use a pink or peachy concealer, depending on skin tone,' says Kay. 'If you are pale, it is common for the under-eye area to be a little blue, so choose a concealer in a pale, peachy colour. If your skin is an olive colour, use a deeper peach shade of concealer to balance the grey. If you have dark skin, use a terracotta shade to counteract the discoloration.'

If you're not a foundation wearer, put concealer over the top of your moisturizer in the places that need evening out

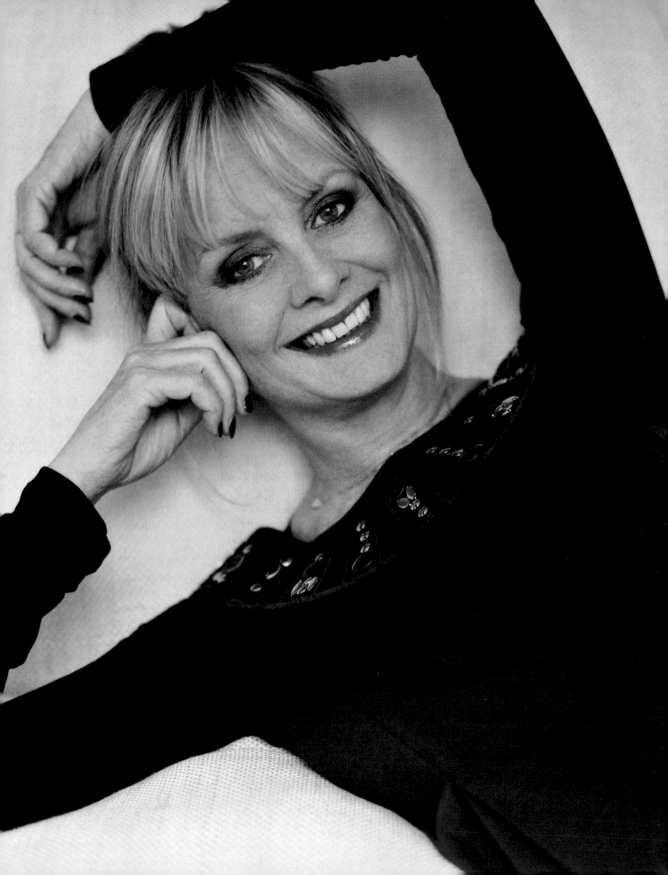

Barbara suggests …

1 **YOUR CONCEALER** should be highly pigmented, creamy and not drying.

2 **YOU SHOULD BE ABLE TO APPLY IT WITH YOUR FINGERTIPS OR A BRUSH** (I often load up a retractable lip brush with it and put it in my bag). You want it to blend easily but, at the same time, conceal.

3 **IF YOU'RE APPLYING ON A LARGE AREA** use your fingers.

4 **IF YOU'RE DOING A PRECISE AREA,** a sun mark on your forehead or a blotch on your cheek, just dab it on with your little brush. A brush is essential for under eyes because even if you're very slim, your fingers won't be small enough to get into the dark shadows.

5 **ON YOUR EYES THE KEY IS TO FILL IN ONLY THE DARK BITS;** if you put concealer over your puffy bags, you'll just draw attention to them. A clever place to put it is on the inner corner of the eye on the bridge of the nose.

6 **CONCEALER IS TERRIFIC ON EYELIDS** as it evens out your tone, also around the base of the nose where skin tends to redden.

7 **ALWAYS PUT IT ON AFTER FOUNDATION OR YOU'LL WIPE IT ALL AWAY.** The colour is obviously very important. Too orange doesn't suit anyone. Choose a concealer the way you'd choose a foundation. I recommend having two: one that's a tad darker for your face, and a slightly paler one for the eye area as your skin tends to be lighter there.

the face

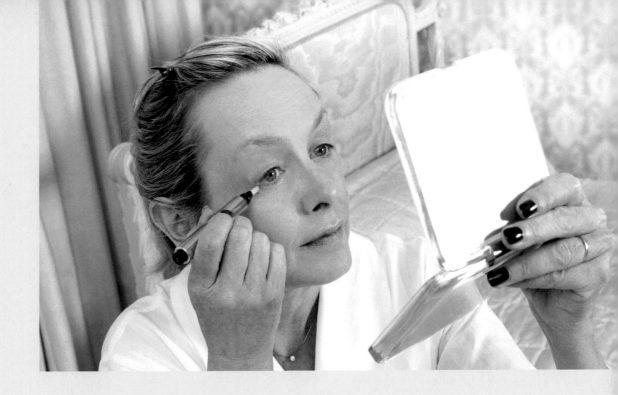

CONCEALERS YOU MIGHT LIKE TO TRY

LUXURY

- *Yves Saint Laurent Touche Éclat Radiant Touch Concealer*
- *Laura Mercier Secret Camouflage (this product is amazing!)*

MIDDLE

- *Bobbi Brown Creamy Concealer*
- *MAC Select Cover-up*

BUDGET

- *Boots No.7 Instant Radiance Concealer*
- *Bourjois D'un Coup de Pinceau Imperfection Corrector*

LIGHT REFLECTORS

THERE ARE TWO WAYS TO USE LIGHT REFLECTORS. One is to bring out bone structure, the other to bring light to anywhere that's looking a little sunken or shadowy. After all, as we know, everything can go south and muscles do begin to sag as we age, which can leave cheeks very hollow.

'Use a little highlighter in that sunken "V" under the cheekbone, or under the lower lip, or anywhere you feel is looking shadowy,' says Barbara. 'To bring out your bone structure, try a peachy shimmer – or gold – and stroke it over the brow bone, cheekbones, the centre of your top eyelid, the "V" of your upper lip and chin tip.'

You might like to try **CHANEL** and **BOURJOIS** blushers. Use these on the cheeks where they can add a bit of bloom and vitality to the face. Colours are suitable for both the palest of pale to dark skins. Another winner for older skins is **REVLON SKINLIGHTS, WARM GLOW** or a similar product.

'It is great on the cheeks if your face is really tired or if you're feeling flat. Apply some of this underneath the blusher and it will add that much-needed vitality to the face,' says Kay.

For a youthful glow, try a peachy shimmer and stroke it over the high spots where the light naturally hits your face

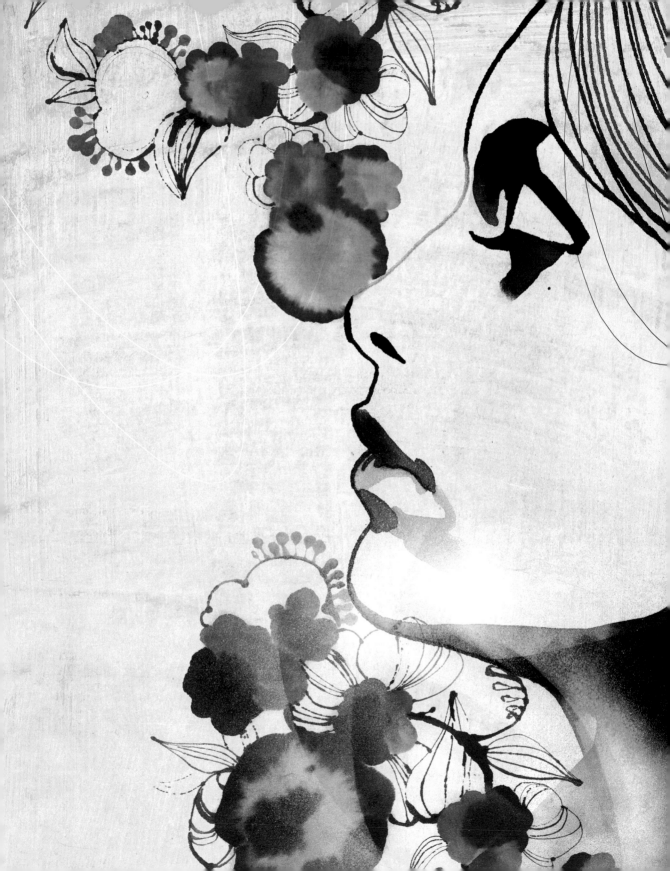

NATURAL AND CRUELTY FREE IS BEST

I'M A BIG BELIEVER IN USING, WHEREVER POSSIBLE, BEAUTY PRODUCTS WITH NO ANIMAL TESTING. I'm a strong believer that this kind of research purely for cosmetics is unacceptable. It's also important to me that you try not to slather your skin with chemicals. Try to look for products that do not have parabens, lanolin, petrochemicals and perfume listed among the ingredients. Nicotine patches work on the basis of being absorbed through the skin, so think carefully about the products you are applying to the face and body. To check the cruelty-free credentials of your cosmetics, go to www.leapingbunny.org.

COLOUR ME BEAUTIFUL

IN THE LATE SIXTIES AND EARLY SEVENTIES, I WAS MAD ABOUT BIBA MAKE-UP. It was created by Barbara Hulanicki. Women and retailers owe her so much for being so ahead of her time and for being so stylish. She is still one of the most beautiful, stylish women I know. I remember the first time I ever saw her at the Abingdon Road Biba store, and thinking how amazing she was. She was the first to bring out make-up colours that included deep purple eyeshadows and black nailpolishes.

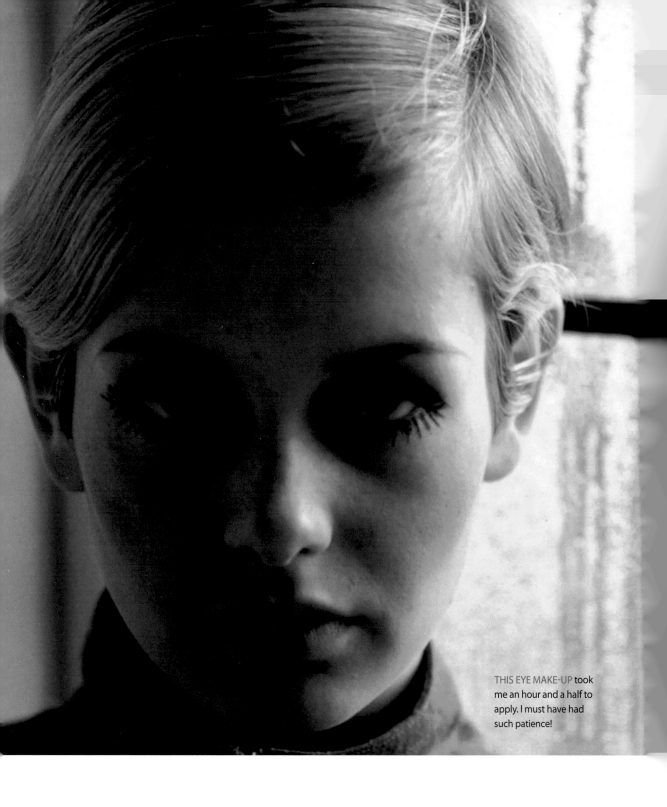

THIS EYE MAKE-UP took me an hour and a half to apply. I must have had such patience!

Make-up can really take years off you if it is properly applied. In general, less is more, but experiment

Barbara Hulanicki did what all the top cosmetics companies are doing today. Go to any big cosmetics store and you can find every single colour of make-up under the sun. Just as there are a myriad choices on the high street for clothes, so there are for make-up. But sometimes too much variety can become overwhelming.

'Too many people give up their own instinct when it comes to make-up, but there is no cosmetic panacea,' says Kay.

And she's right. There's no rule that says you can't still use colour for effect; just don't overdo it.

'Go for a flash of colour rather than anything more. The main thing is to get the skin looking right first.'

There's no need to be scared of colour, just because you are older. The trick is to modify the way you use it. What's more, according to Barbara Daly, there's no rule about what colour suits what type of skin.

'The only rule is the contrast rule. The paler your skin, the more contrasty anything looks that you put against it. So, say you were going for a mid-grey to get smokey eyes, on pale skin it will look quite dark, whereas on olive skin it won't. The darker the colour, the paler the skin, the stronger it will look.'

Barbara suggests that instead of covering your whole lid with colour, use a neutral eye-shadow and then use a brighter colour as eyeliner. That way, you can still have some fun without drawing attention to any creases in your lids. For make-up artist Bobbi Brown, it's about wearing the right colours.

'We lose our natural colouring as we age, so the trick is to use make-up to add that colour back,' says Bobbi. 'You want to use shades that brighten up the face. Too much make-up can add years to your face, as well as look mask-like and unnatural. Make-up should always enhance your features, not overpower them, especially now, so use an extra-light hand. You can always add more if need be, but it's far more difficult to take it away if there is too much.'

Above all, muck around, have fun at home, experiment, try new techniques and shades. Don't be frightened. **BE BRAVE!**

TREATS AND SERUMS

THERE'S NOTHING MORE FUN THAN HAVING A GIRLY NIGHT IN, PUTTING ON A FACE MASK AND RELAXING EITHER WITH A GOOD BOOK OR IN FRONT OF THE TELLY. Masks are a great way to give your skin an extra treat – whether it's a boost of moisture or vitamins, or skin sloughing.

Another great way to give your skin a boost is through serums. These magic potions are packed with super-high concentrations of the active ingredients that protect, heal and help skin repair and rebuild itself. They can also be customized to your needs at the time: whether it's lightening and clarifying, ultra-moisturizing or energizing.

the face

TREATS YOU MIGHT LIKE TO TRY

(although olive oil and honey can be just as good!)

1 Serum

LUXURY

- *Estée Lauder Advanced Night Repair Protective Recovery Complex*
- *Zelens Skin Science Radical Defense Serum*

MIDDLE

- *Dr. Andrew Weil for Origins™ Mega-Mushroom Face Serum*

BUDGET

- *Boots No. 7 Protect and Perfect Beauty Serum*

2 Skin Sloughing

LUXURY

- *Elemis Papaya Enzyme Peel*

MIDDLE

- *Kiehl's Overnight Biological Peel*

BUDGET

- *Avon ANEW Clinical Advanced Dermabrasion System*

3 Masks

LUXURY

- *Amanda Lacey Restoring Mandarin Mask*
- *Dr Alkaitis Organic Universal Mask*

MIDDLE

- *Jurlique Moisture Replenishing Mask*
- *Bliss Triple Oxygen Instant Energizing Mask*

BUDGET

- *Dr Hauschka Rejuvenating Mask*
- *Liz Earle Naturally Active Skincare Intensive Nourishing Treatment*

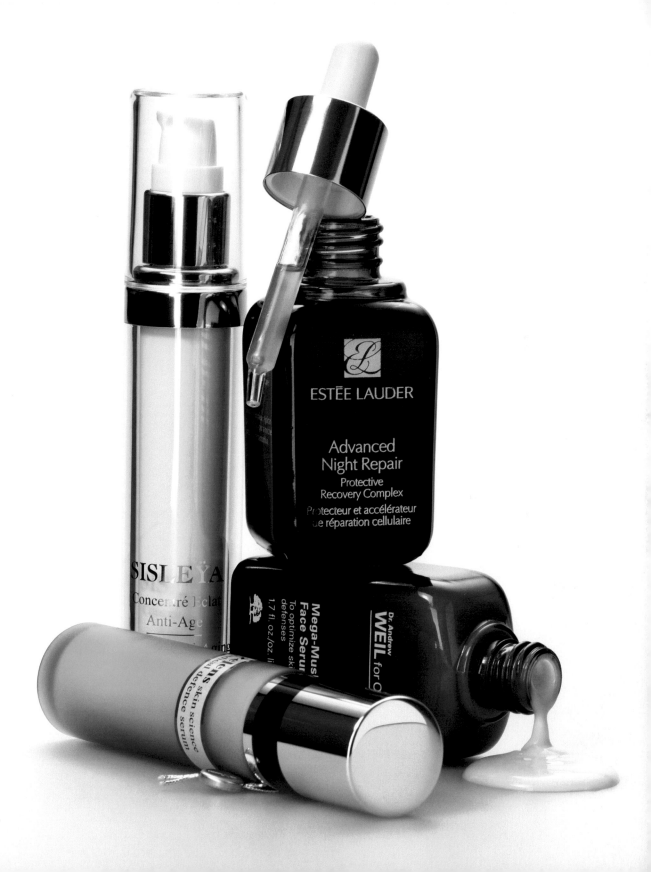

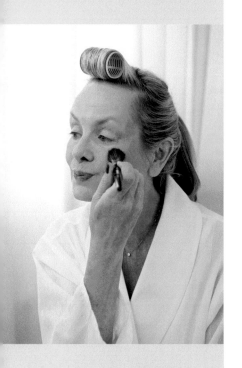

BLUSHER

IF USING A MATT POWDER BLUSHER, APPLY WITH A LARGE, SOFT BRUSH, JUST DUSTING OVER THE CHEEK GENTLY. Don't overdo it. Also be careful with brownish powder shades down the side of the cheekbones. This can look really dated and is very ageing. Unless you have very dark skin, a soft pinkish hue on the cheek looks much more natural. Tip: when applying, smile and dust blusher gently on cheeks. Barbara advises that everyone should have a wardrobe of blushers. At different times of year, you need different shades.

'A little bit warmer and more reddish for use on a winter's night, when you're wearing darker colours; a nice peachy/apricot colour for summertime. Also, invest in a classic, pinky rose. It's the nearest thing to natural and works for almost every skin type.'

When you blush, blood comes to the surface of your skin, making it pink-red. Forget about trying to copy shades as you're told to do in magazines; the whole point about blusher is in using it to make your skin look good and your eyes bright and healthy.

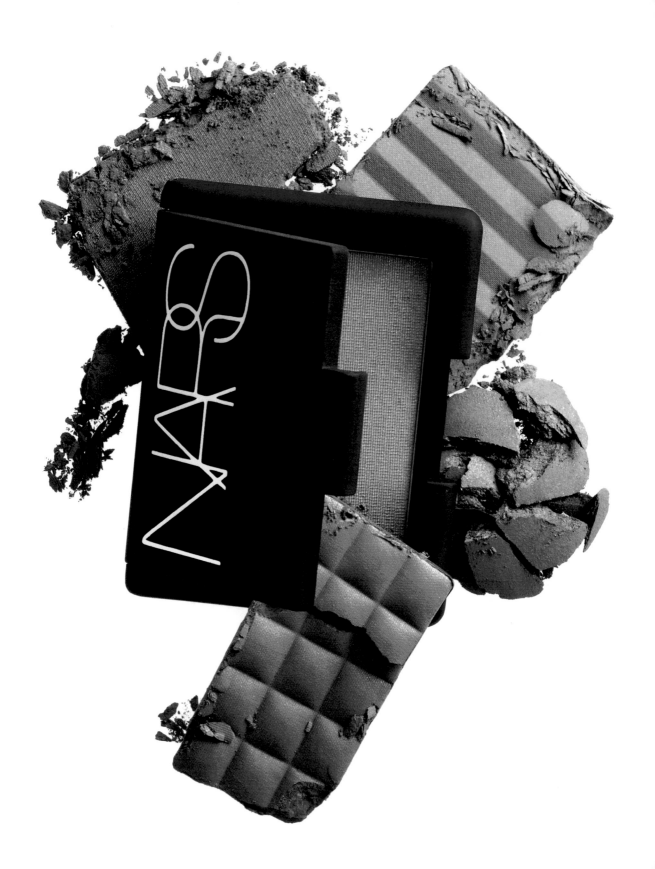

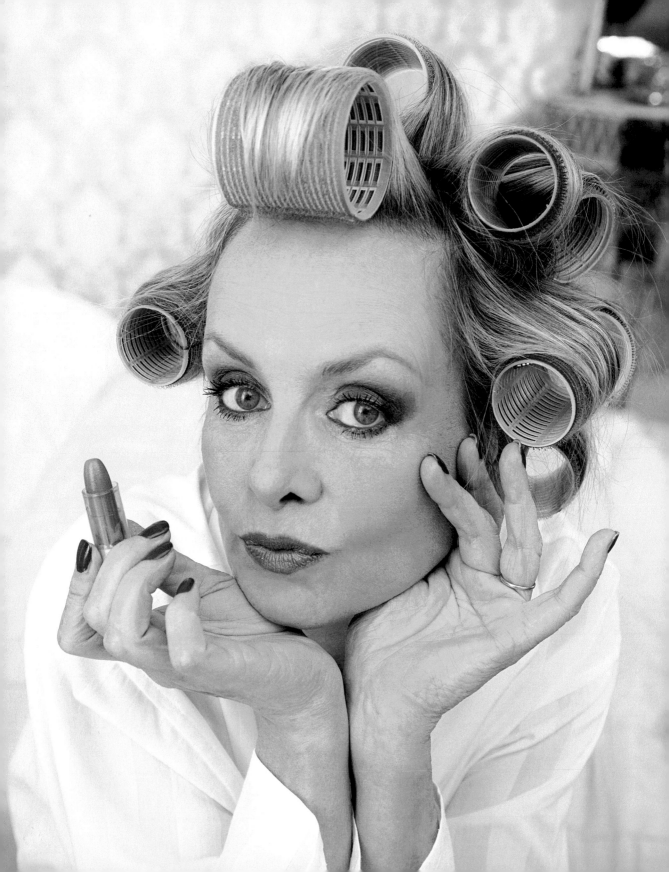

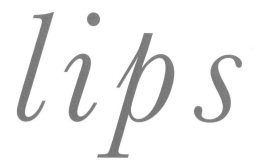

lips

ONE OF THE SIDE EFFECTS OF AGEING CAN BE THAT LIPS START TO THIN. This can become even more pronounced if you have been (or still are) a smoker.

'Invest in a treatment lip balm or gloss that uses lip-plumping peptides and hyaluronic acid, which occurs in the skin naturally and holds up to a thousand times its weight in water,' suggests Antonia Wyatt.

If you want some extra shine or moisture, I think it's safest to find a lipstick in a mid-tone then put a little gloss on top. If you want darker or red lips, apply the darker colour to the inside of the lips only, on top of a more neutral shade. Blend gently but avoid the darker colour reaching the lip edges as you may then get feathering. Also be careful of sheer lipsticks as they have more wax and tend to melt at skin temperature.

'If you want to stop feathering, those long-stay lipsticks really do stay put,' says Barbara Daly. 'Also, lip pencils help. Put a little powder round the edge of your mouth and gently fill in with lip pencil. Feathering is going to happen, so do remember: the darker the lipstick, the more it will show.'

A little dab of illuminator at the bow of the lip is a nice effect for evening. Put on before lip liner and lipstick and it gives instant pout.

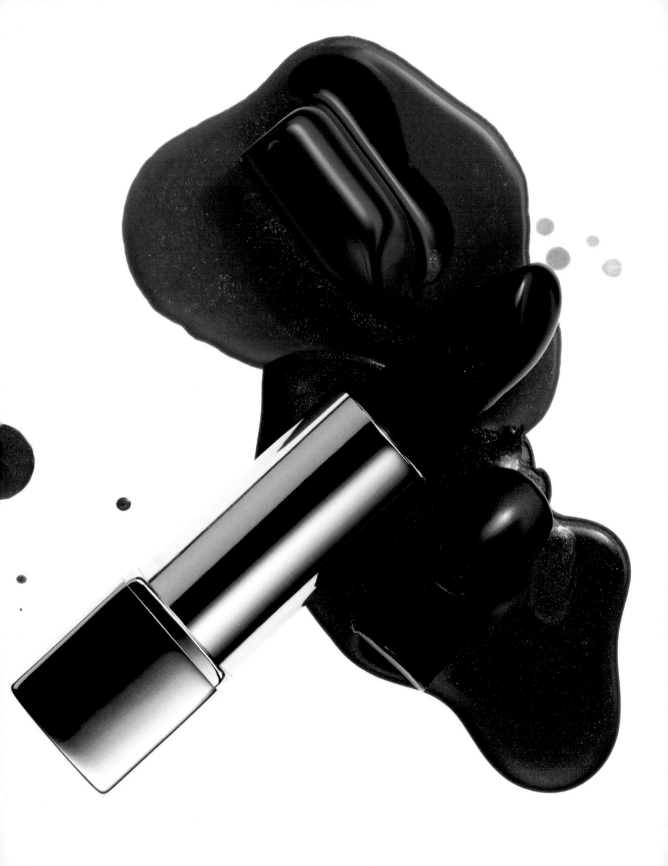

LIP PRODUCTS YOU MIGHT LIKE TO TRY

1 Lipsticks

LUXURY

- *Chanel Rouge Hydrabase containing shea butter*

MIDDLE

- *Lancôme Le Rouge Absolu*

BUDGET

- *Max Factor Lipfinity*

2 Lip liners

LUXURY

- *NARS Lipliner Pencil*
- *Sisley Phyto-Lèvres Perfect Lipliner*

MIDDLE

- *Clinique Quickliner for Lips*

BUDGET

- *Jemma Kidd Shape and Shade Lip Liner and Lip Fill*

3 Lip balms

LUXURY

- *By Terry Baume de Rose SPF 15 Lip Care*

MIDDLE

- *Elizabeth Arden Eight Hour Cream*
- *Shiseido Benefiance Full Correction Lip Treatment*

BUDGET

- *Dr. Andrew Weil for Origins™ Conditioning Lip Balm with Turmeric*
- *Kiehl's Lip Balm #1*

MAKE-UP SIN BIN

A few techniques to avoid

1 **APPLYING YOUR MAKE-UP IN ARTIFICIAL LIGHT,** unless you have professional make-up lights. Even then, natural is best.

2 **FROSTED PEARLY LIPSTICKS.** They make your lips look old, old, old!

3 **STRONG EYES AND BRIGHT LIPS AT THE SAME TIME.** This is a big no-no. One or the other will suffice.

4 **OVERDOING EYEBROW PENCIL.** Go easy or you'll end up looking like a transvestite!

5 **SHIMMERING EYESHADOWS.** They can seek out the crepe and showcase it!

6 **HEAVY FOUNDATIONS.** Ignore their claim to cover wrinkles. They won't.

7 **IF YOU CAN REMEMBER WITH GREAT AFFECTION** the make-up look from the first time round, twenty-odd years ago, it's not for you: it was your look of the time, so move on.

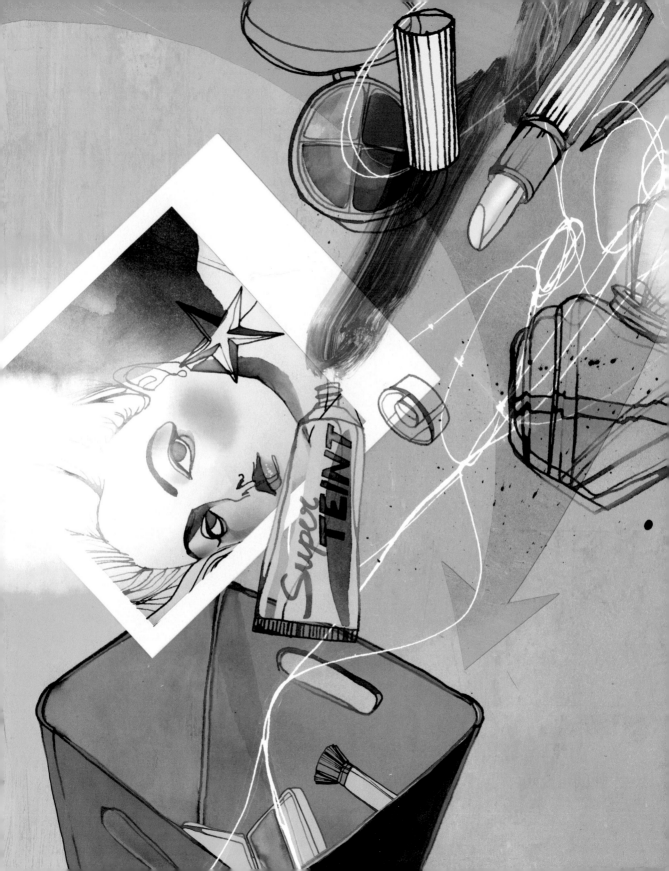

neck
&décolletage

IF YOU ARE INCLUDING YOUR NECK IN YOUR DAILY BEAUTY ROUTINE, THERE IS NOTHING TO WORRY ABOUT HERE. However, many women forget how vital it is to continue cream down to the décolletage. I don't do special neck exercises but when I do a Pilates class, obviously the neck area does get included. For many women, the skin can slacken in this area. As you age, the neck muscle starts pulling downwards, creating what can best be described as a turkey neck. Using a good neck cream with upwards massaging movements will superficially plump and smooth, and there are lots of neck creams and treatments on the market. But if the look of your neck is really bothering you, try acupuncture. It can actually increase the tone of the muscle and give a bit of a lift.

You might like to try more intense treatments like radio frequency or Thermage. These (although some say Thermage can be quite painful) work deep down below the skin's surface to lift and tighten sagging necks and jawlines. I recently tried radio frequency, a treatment which kick-starts everything into action, tightening muscles and stimulating collagen production. I found it worked wonders on my tummy area.

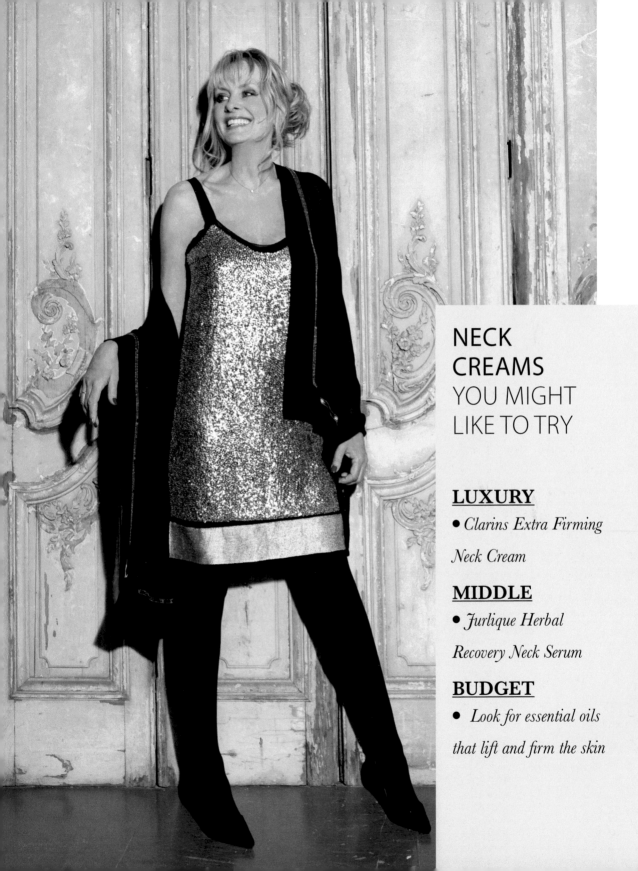

NECK CREAMS
YOU MIGHT LIKE TO TRY

LUXURY
• *Clarins Extra Firming Neck Cream*

MIDDLE
• *Jurlique Herbal Recovery Neck Serum*

BUDGET
• *Look for essential oils that lift and firm the skin*

cosmetic surgery

IT IS IMPOSSIBLE TO IGNORE COSMETIC DERMATOLOGY AND SURGERY. IT'S HAPPENING ALL AROUND US, ON OUR TELEVISION SCREENS, IN MAGAZINES AND, OF COURSE, AMONG OUR FRIENDS.

But if you're not keen on the idea of undergoing general anaesthetic, there are now plenty of options available to women without having to go under the knife. In fact the trend is moving more towards tweaking and enhancing and away from that wind-tunnel face-lift look. But, if you do choose to have cosmetic surgery, select your doctor carefully, either through recommendation or by checking with the **BRITISH ASSOCIATION OF AESTHETIC PLASTIC SURGEONS**. Ask all the questions you need to and, most importantly, ask to see pictures of their work up close. Don't go for a cheap alternative. These are operations after all – so there will always be a risk. If done well and with subtlety, it certainly seems to give some people confidence. It's a very personal choice.

NON-INVASIVE PROCEDURES & LASERS

I TALKED TO BEAUTY EDITOR AND CONSULTANT ANTONIA WHYATT ABOUT THE LATEST TREATMENTS AVAILABLE SHOULD YOU WISH TO CONSIDER SOMETHING MORE THAN SKIN DEEP. Before you do anything like this, as with cosmetic surgery, contact the **BRITISH ASSOCIATION OF DERMATOLOGISTS** to check up on the qualifications of your chosen dermatologist, and the **BRITISH ASSOCIATION OF AESTHETIC PLASTIC SURGEONS**, as many laser experts will be aesthetic surgeons. Ask the doctor how many of these procedures they have performed. The more the better, as practice makes perfect. 'You don't want lasers to be a doctor's sideline, you want it to be one of their main focuses.' Antonia recommends that laser procedures are carried out during wintertime ideally, when the skin is pale and the sun is weak. For a couple of months, avoid the sun after the skin has been resurfaced, as you will have lost the natural defence of the outer layer of dead skin cells. You will have to be rigorous about wearing sun screen for a few weeks and staying out of the sun. Beware of dermatologists who have bought the expensive equipment (laser machines cost around £150,000) and are just trying to use it to pay it off. Always have a consultation first and get two opinions.

'Our skin is a road map to the lives we've lived: too much sunbathing as a teenager (brown spots, freckles), lots of time spent outdoors (broken veins), babies (brown patches, skin tags, eye bags),' says Antonia. 'While there's a lot we can do on the pampering front to make ourselves look and feel our best, if you really want to take it a step further, lasers are the new non-invasive solution for sun-damaged, lacklustre skin that has lost its plumpness.'

With the new generation of lasers it takes around two days for the skin to recover. 'It depends on the intensities used, but it's typically forty-eight hours,' says Dr Neil Walker, one of the UK's top dermatologists and laser experts. 'Sometimes it can be significantly longer.' So once again check with your doctor, ask questions. No one's going to bite your head off.

the face

Here are Antonia's recommendations

Lasers are good for tightening sagging skin on jaws, under the chin, on necks and tummies

1. Fraxel

On the face, neck and décolletage Fraxel is one of the new lasers that dermatologists rave about for evening out skin tone and plumping fine lines. It has minimal recovery time (one to three days of looking a bit sunburned), and works on the surface of your skin. Instead of one beam, it has lots of tiny ones that resurface your skin little by little. Think of your skin as a pixellated painting and the Fraxel (helped by a computer) fixes and smooths all the colours to become an even tone. At the same time, the energy of the laser on the way down stimulates skin-plumping collagen (literally the building blocks that make our skin full). The treatment is divided into three sessions and the results last for two to three years.

Fraxel is pretty uncomfortable as it feels like lots of little needles pulsating into your face. The therapist will put on a gel to help numb you, but this is only mildly effective. The treatment takes about twenty minutes, and afterwards your skin is likely to feel wind-burned.

2. Titan

Titan is another popular laser. It has a single beam that penetrates deeply and uses infrared heat to stimulate collagen renewal. After a couple of sessions the jaw and neck start to firm up due to all that stimulation, which carries on for between three and six months after the treatment. Other lasers that do this are Thermage and Emax.

The intensity of the treatment depends on your pain threshold, and the doctor can adjust the laser for this so let them know how you're feeling. This is not pain-free by any means but is supposed to be the least painful of the intense laser treatments. Afterwards your skin will be red but not swollen or burned-looking.

3. IPL and peels

Antonia says the best way to remove age spots is with IPL (intense pulse laser). This targets the pigment and gently zaps it off the surface of the skin. A less expensive way is to consider Environ's at-home kit, **EVENESCENCE CLARIFYING PATCHES.** These can literally be stuck on stubborn brown spots to both stop melanin production (the stuff that makes them brown) and lighten them up.

Acid peels can be another brilliant way to refresh the skin and get rid of superficial sun damage. They sound terrifying, but actually many of them use fruit acids or glycolic acid to eat away the dead skin cells on top of the skin, revealing fresher, younger skin underneath. These do not have to be too strong to give nice results in the dermatologist's office. At-home peels can help keep your skin cells turning over (this slows down greatly with age), which in turn keeps skin clear, unclogged, and stops any breakouts or dullness. Antonia recommends **DR DENNIS GROSS'S MD SKINCARE ALPHA BETA DAILY FACE PEEL.**

IPL really doesn't hurt, it just feels like warm, concentrated sunlight on your face. Peels can sting and burn, so if it's your first time make sure you let the doctor know and have a light peel. The good news is that the treatment only lasts a few minutes. At Dr David Colbert's in New York you're given a little hand-held fan to blow cool air on your face during the peel.

4. Ingredients to know about

As lines get deeper, one of the most effective anti-ageing skincare ingredients are peptides. Developed for healing wounds, these tiny protein fractions fight wrinkles in two ways. First, they can send specific messages to different cells telling them to build collagen and turn over dead skin cells. Secondly, they slow down the nerve signals sent to the muscles that cause expression lines. Argirelene is a peptide that has a Botox-like effect, in a cream.

the face

Antioxidants: look for these in your creams and serums. They come in many forms, from Vitamins C and E, to green tea and reservatrol (from grapes). They fight ageing by neutralizing cell-destroying free radicals, which are molecules with unstable energy.

TACKLING SPIDER VEINS

MANY OF US DEVELOP RED VEINS AS WE GET OLDER. THIS IS BECAUSE, WITH AGE, THE CUSHIONING LAYER IN YOUR SKIN LOSES ITS PADDING AND ELASTICITY, SO VEINS COME TO THE SURFACE. For little red veins around the nose, a diolite or 'green laser' will zap them. A wavelength of light finds the vein, heats it up and destroys it. Veins will disappear within a week. One of the UK's leading dermatologists and laser experts, Dr Neil Walker, also recommends **VEINWAVE**. This uses an ultra-fine needle to apply heat and high-frequency energy pulses onto the damaged veins, dissolving them. He also suggests a good topical retinoid cream (a mild form of vitamin A, the only FDA-approved wrinkle-buster) to help rebuild collagen.

MOLES

ANTONIA SAYS THAT EVERYONE SHOULD HAVE A SKIN-CANCER CHECK ONCE A YEAR AND I DO. I am quite fair skinned and have freckles, so being checked is vital for me. You want to watch moles that have irregular borders or colour, or are larger than the tip of a pencil rubber. You should always look for changes. Your back is a hard place to check because you can't see it, so when you are shopping take advantage of three-way dressing room mirrors to give yourself a thorough look. The scalp is a hard place to check too, so ask your hairdresser to keep an eye out.

You could try the **MOLE CLINIC (www.themoleclinic.co.uk)**, where they have all the latest equipment and will keep all of your information on file. If they see a suspicious mole, they can now do 'digital mole mapping', whereby they capture high-resolution images of your whole body, then do it again on a return visit so they can compare the size of all the moles.

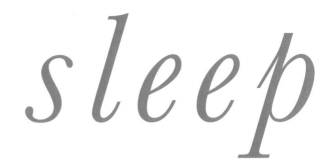

sleep

A GOOD NIGHT'S SLEEP LEAVES US FEELING RESTED, REVIVED AND FULL OF BEANS. IT IS, WITHOUT QUESTION, ONE OF THE BEST THINGS YOU CAN DO TO HELP YOU FEEL GOOD AND MAKE YOU LOOK BETTER.

I love my sleep. I'm the big sleeper of the world. It's probably one of my saving graces. I can sleep through most things. At night, that is. I have never been able to get to grips with siestas. I know an actress who can even go to sleep in the make-up chair! I can't do that. I like eight and a half to nine hours every night if I can manage it.

If you're more of a night owl, try what my friend does after lunch to recharge. The important thing, she says, is to lie down somewhere that's not your bed. If you cat nap in your own bed, you may fall too deeply asleep and wake up groggy.

Here's what she does

● Lie on the floor on your back, legs stretched out in front of you, head on a cushion, placing your hands on your tummy.
● In one of your hands, hold a pencil upright.
● Close your eyes and relax.
● When the pencil drops, it will wake you up, reviving and recharging you just enough to get through the rest of your day.

the face

NIGHT CREAMS
YOU MIGHT LIKE TO TRY

LUXURY

- *Estée Lauder Re-Nutriv Re-Creation Night Creme*

MIDDLE

- *Caudalie Vinoperfect Radiance Serum Complexion Correcting*
- *Organic Pharmacy Antioxidant Face Firming Serum*
- *RoC Retin-Ox Intensive Anti-wrinkle Night Cream*

BUDGET

- *Weleda Wild Rose Night Cream*

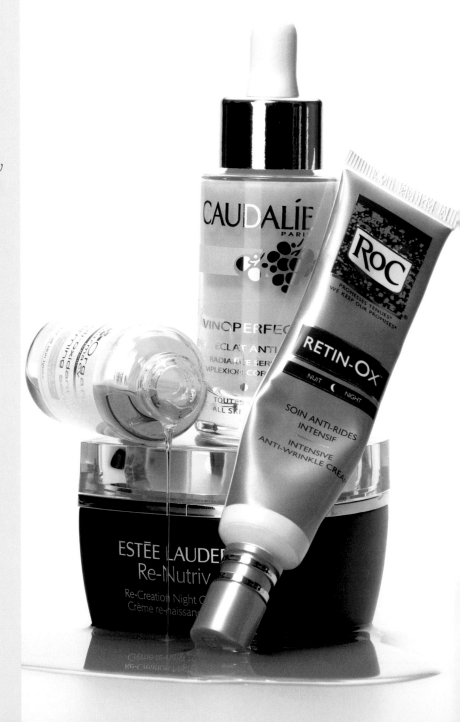

Sleep is all about regeneration. Alongside a good rest, one of the cheapest and best ways to stay looking healthy is to drink water. Two pints a day are recommended, which I find hard sometimes, but at the very least try to drink a big glass of water first thing in the morning on waking, and last thing at night before you go to sleep. It makes such a difference. I know, it might make you pee in the night, but it's worth it! Better still, try to have that night-time glug an hour before bedtime. On waking, some people swear by hot water with a slice of lemon to kick-start your system. Or add to that some fresh ginger – it's lovely.

'When you sleep your body releases growth hormones,' says Tony Vargas, Vice President of Research and Development at Elizabeth Arden. 'When you're a kid that makes you grow; when you're an adult that turns into maintenance and repair mode. While sleeping, skin expels toxins and gets busy with building collagen and creating new cells.'

This is why lack of sleep can cause you to look grey and pasty. Also, the worse the sleep, the less blood circulation to your skin, which can lead to dark circles under the eyes. Layer on top of this the anxiety insomnia causes (frown lines), and you see how important sleep is for you to feel, and therefore look, good.

Temperature is very important for a good night's sleep. I prefer it cooler rather than too warm. In the summer, I like the window open. In the winter, although the heat is off, I just snuggle under the duvet to keep warm and nearly always wear winceyette PJs, which I love. Why is it they make you feel so secure?

I find reading a book just before I go to sleep really helps. It slowly allows the mind to wind down, distracting it from any worries. Setting yourself a wind-down routine really helps. Also, it's worth remembering that although alcohol can send you to sleep, it's only sedating you and you'll wake up five hours later, when your blood-sugar level spikes.

At night, I always moisturize intensely with a rich cream. If my skin feels extra dry, I'll add a thin film of vitamin E oil. Recently I have even been applying Vaseline around the eye bone and face. This works for me, but your skin may be dramatically different.

the face

83

hair

EVER SINCE THE AGE OF SIXTEEN, I HAVE HAD BLONDE HIGHLIGHTS. MY NATURAL HAIR COLOUR IS MOUSY BROWN SO IF I WANTED I COULD EXPERIMENT WITH LOTS OF DIFFERENT COLOURS, BUT I'M NOT BRAVE ENOUGH. I LOVE BEING BLONDE. It's too much a part of who I am for me to change it now. Often when I think, Oh God, I look dowdy, it's because I need the highlights doing. A trip to the hairdresser can be so transforming, not only for your mood, but for its ability to add a level of elegance to the overall vision of a woman, regardless of what we're doing, wearing, feeling. It can also boost your confidence. If you look good, you feel good! Hairdressers love nothing better than making a customer feel a million times more gorgeous as they walk out of the door.

If you're feeling like a new look, I wouldn't be so bold as to suggest purple stripes or to shave your head. But I do think it's worth seeking out a fabulous hair salon with a good reputation and splurging on a cut and/or colour. It's so important to do your research, especially with colour. We've all seen the disasters of a bad dye job.

For years there's been an unwritten rule that suggests you shouldn't have long hair when you get past a certain age. Poppycock! Unfortunately, some women make the mistake of going to the opposite extreme and hacking it all off. Don't! Unless you have strong features, too-short hair can be harsh and a lost opportunity to add softness to your features. It's impossible to generalize, but for me a fringe softens everything. It is also a clever tool to conceal the inevitable lines. A few layers around the face can also be flattering.

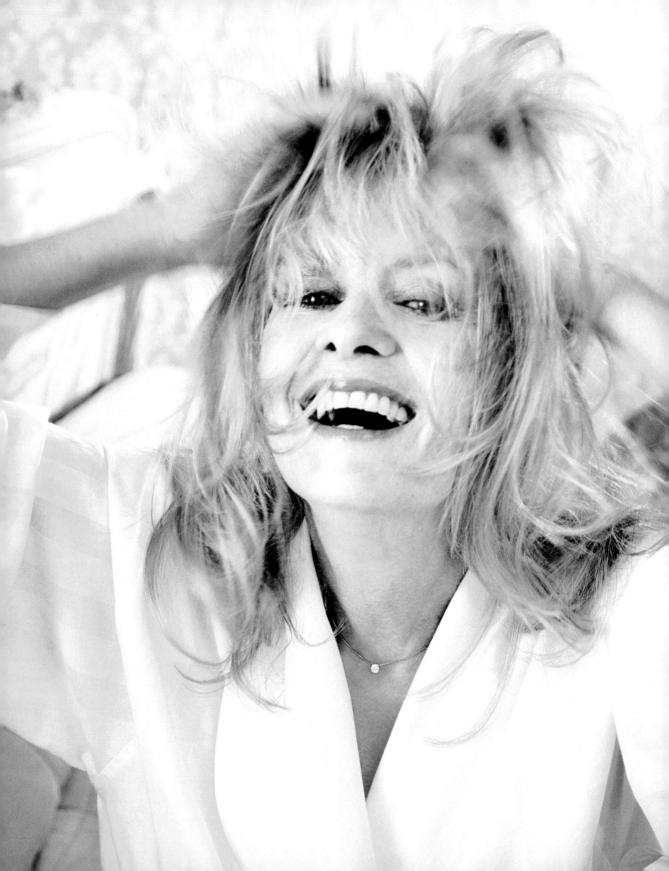

Treating yourself to a good cut and colour is the best investment in your appearance you can make

I find longer hair easier for me to do on a daily basis. I can wash it, dry it, put it in big hot rollers for ten minutes, then put it up in a ponytail or chignon, or leave it down. Whenever I have cut my hair shorter, it has always required more styling.

From the fateful day in 1966 that colourist Daniel Galvin and Leonard, at Leonard's hairdressing salon, gave me the little blonde crop that launched me, I have had blonde highlights. I get so many letters about where I get my hair done. It started off at House of Leonard in Mayfair. Daniel Galvin coloured my hair brilliantly with highlights and continued to do so for many years. Then his son Daniel Junior took over. Daniel Junior moved to Michaeljohn, another fab salon, so I followed him there. Over the last few years I've had the brilliant attention of Poppy, Mandy, Steve and Lee, the colourists at Michaeljohn who are excellent. When I'm in New York, I go to John Frieda. John Frieda, aged sixteen, used to wash my hair at Leonard's when I was eighteen. Now he's one of the most successful hairdressers in the world. Happily, we've stayed friends and it's lovely to bring it full circle. All of these salons are great. As well as having your hair coloured, it's so important to keep your hair in good order with a professional cut every few weeks. Fred at Michaeljohn cuts mine and Matthew Wade styles it brilliantly for photo shoots.

I can't profess to be the expert on other hair colour. Lester Baldwin, hair colourist for the last forty years and a permanent fixture at John Frieda's London salon, is one of my hair experts.

HAIR PRODUCTS
YOU MIGHT LIKE TO TRY

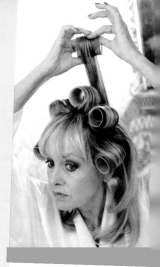

1 Anti-ageing

- *Kerastase Age Recharge – an entire anti-ageing line*
- *Frederic Fekkai Advanced Haircare Ageless Shampoo*

2 Hairbrushes

Try to get natural bristle – it doesn't tear hair. Start brushing hair at the tangled ends when it's wet and supple, working your way up rather than pulling the knots from the top into dry, fragile ends. Mason Pearson are still my favourites.

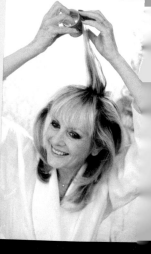

3 Conditioners

It's great to use a conditioner to keep your ends from going brassy or bleaching out. Try John Frieda or Aveda colour conditioners.

4 Serums

- *Bumble and bumble Treatment range*
- *John Frieda Overnight Repair Serum*

5 Conditioners

- *Philip Kingsley Elasticizer*
- *James Brown London Moisture Mask for Hair*

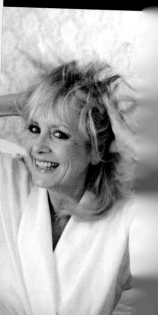

'It would be nice if we lived in a society based on not how you look. But we do, and the plus in the twenty-first century is there are so many great places to go and have a cut and colour,' he says. 'Treating yourself to this is a fantastic investment and can work miracles towards building up confidence levels and generally making you feel good about yourself.'

AND WHY NOT?

'How we feel about ourselves is inextricably linked to looking good. Hair is one area which, with a bit of help from the experts, can improve your appearance on a multitude of levels.'

So go on, treat yourself. I know ladies who go weekly to the hairdressers. I go about every six weeks, when my highlights need doing.

THE GREY AREA

MY NATURAL HAIR COLOUR IS MOUSE, BUT LOTS OF WOMEN GO GREY, SOME AS YOUNG AS TWENTY. About one in ten women who go grey can do so and carry it off well. This is down to the vitality of the skin tone, the eye colour, the shape of the haircut and a woman's confidence, in equal measure. Women with lovely flinty-blue eyes suit grey especially. As we grow older, we lose natural colour in our skin tone, eyes and lips. Grey hair is nature's way of softening our hair colour.

'Fabulous silver-fox colour can look chic and elegant as long as hair is kept in optimum condition,' says Daniel Galvin. 'When your colourist achieves the perfect colour for you, the first thing people will notice is the colour of your eyes, not your hair!' Skin will look refreshed and eyes will sparkle when your hair colour is right.'

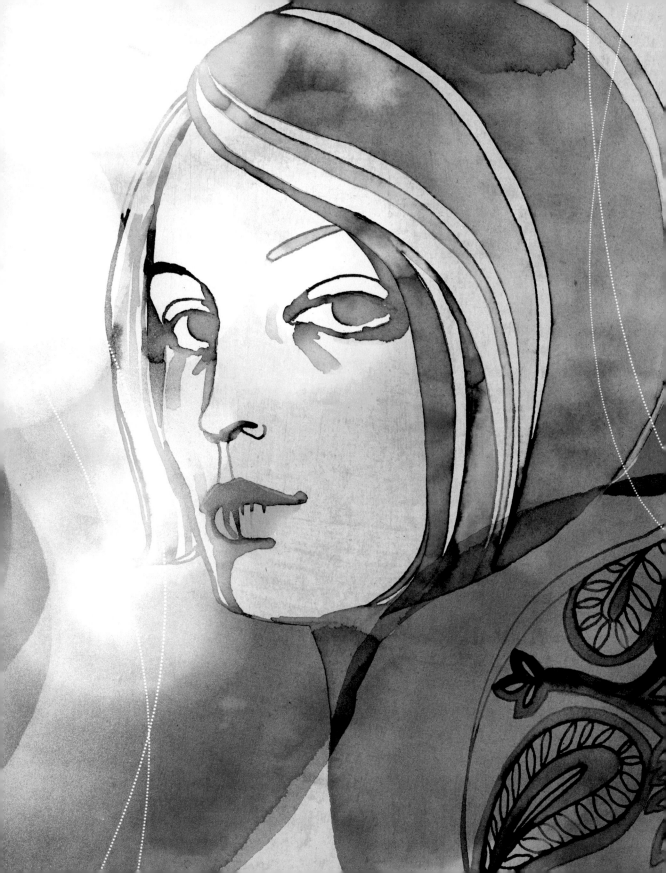

Moisturizing products become more essential with grey hair

Daniel has long been an advocate of the bottle before the knife. Most hair salons worth their salt will have a chat with a new customer to talk about how far they want to go by way of tints or lights.

'For our older customers, we would usually suggest tinting to add depth, pigment and thickness to naturally grey hair,' Lester says. Grey can become a little bit watery and translucent. The cut you choose has a more solid base to work from when grey hair has been tinted. Also, grey tends to go wiry. It can be a bit of a shock for women who previously might have had much smoother hair texture. For a while, as the grey takes over, there can be two textures of hair going on at the same time.

GOING THE WHOLE WAY

IF YOU ARE GOING TO EMBRACE YOUR GREY AND SILVER HAIR, familiarize yourself with anti-frizz products, as often it's the texture rather than length or thickness that can be a challenge. There's no rule that says grey isn't gorgeous, nor is there a rule that says colouring your hair is undignified. Go for whatever makes you feel fantastic.

'For me, grey hair is the Jil Sander of hair,' says hair colourist Josh Wood of Real Hair. 'It's slightly austere and out there, but a real statement if you feel psychologically confident enough to pull it off.' For Josh, the key is that the cut has to be very simple. 'It can't be overstyled and the hair has to be in great condition.'

As you age, the hair goes grey and becomes watery and finer as you lose the colour

But don't let your eyebrows become grey: that can be very ageing. As Barbara Daly points out, it's the way she and most make-up artists age people on film sets. Instead, keep them your pre-grey colour.

TOP TIPS ON HAIR COLOURING FOR NATURAL GREYS

1. Blonde

When you are younger and naturally blonde, you have highlights and lowlights to enhance the colour. As you age, the hair goes grey and becomes watery and finer as you lose the colour. To keep the hair completely blonde you must start filling in the hair around the highlights, putting a tint between the foils. This acts as an artificial base, covering the grey, to which the highlights are added. This is easy to do, and essentially, as you age, it is fairly easy staying blonde.

Don't go too ash, instead opt for a multi-tonal effect, keeping your own soft grey as the lightest highlight, contrasting subtly with warmer honey-blondes.

2. Brunette

The good thing about wanting to stay brunette is that hair technology enables women to keep the hair a much

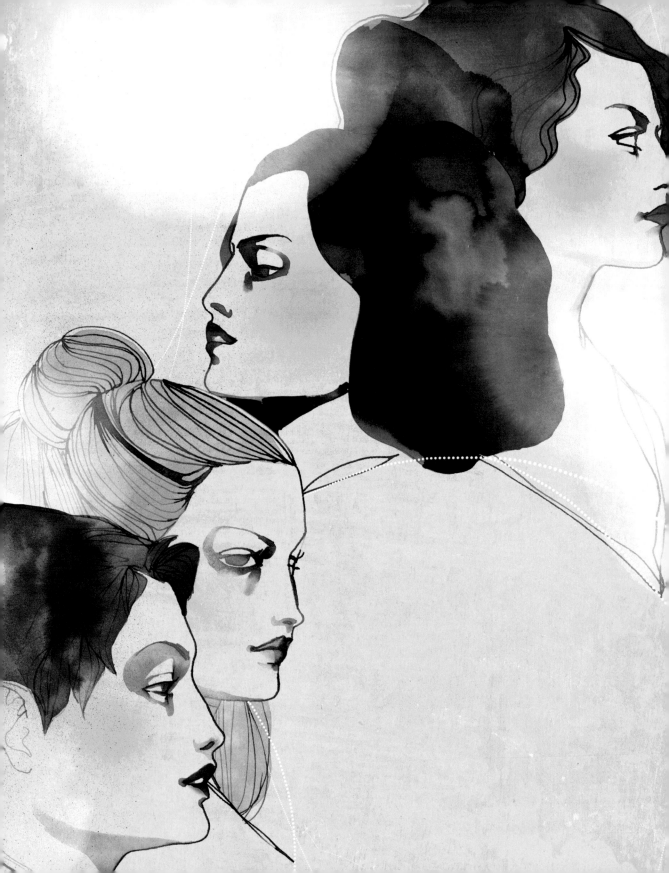

younger colour and still look natural. It is very easy to stay darker for longer. However, the downside is that your roots will give you away as the grey shows through. To counteract this, be alert to your hair styling and avoid centre partings, warns Lester. Don't be tempted to go too dark, says Daniel. 'Soften brunettes with some rich reverse lights to create movement through the hair. In between salon visits have a vegetable colour to maintain depth of colour and enhance shine,' he suggests.

3. Black
Unless you are a goth through and through, don't keep dyeing your hair black as you will look like a member of the Addams Family. Change your shade to dark brown instead. You will look warmer and younger.

4. Red
Until your forties, be as red as you want. As you get older, go for softer shades such as apricot or strawberry; these are warmer and more natural. Hair will naturally fade as we grow older so do not attempt to recapture the red of your youth. Soften with lights and a vegetable colour for gorgeous, shiny healthy hair.

5. Shocking pink
If you are a bit of a rebel, there's nothing that says you shouldn't continue a punk approach to hair colouring as you get older. I know a few women who dye their hair bright pink, crimson red and bright orange. Granarchy in the UK! Great. The only thing to factor in is that bright colours can be harsh and unkind.

BLOW-DRY

AS MY HAIR EXPERTS SAY, IF YOUR HAIR IS IN GREAT CONDITION AND YOU HAVE A CUT THAT SUITS YOUR FACE SHAPE, hair can look glamorous and sexy at any length. A weekly blow-dry may seem extravagant, but it doesn't have to cost a bomb and is the best way to help keep hair looking groomed. Think of it as an investment in 'you' time, and if you haven't got the budget, try it at home.

Here are some tips to make your blow dry last . . .

1 SIT ON YOUR HANDS IF YOU HAVE TO, but running them through your hair will weigh it down with dirt and grease and make it lose shape and volume.

2 HAVE SOME DRY SHAMPOO HANDY, like BUMBLE AND BUMBLE HAIR POWDER or KLORANE, and spray in the roots the morning after or before going out, to absorb grease.

3 SLEEP ON A SATIN PILLOWCASE. It stops hair snagging. It's also good for stopping wrinkles round the eyes.

4 IF YOU HAVE A FRINGE, you can make hair look fresh again by washing and blow-drying the fringe rather than your whole head.

5 RUN OVER ANY BITS that have pouffed out with a hair-straightener and you'll look instantly glamorous again.

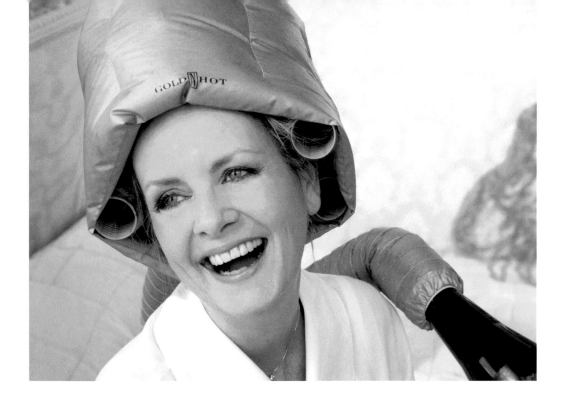

Once in a while it is a good idea to invest in an in-salon deep-conditioning treatment; your hair will thank you for it. Look for Kerastase treatments (**www.kerastase.co.uk**). Salons will tailor them to your hair type. These put conditioners and strengtheners into each hair's internal shaft. Biolustre (biolustre.com) is painted onto hair and hardens under heat for an hour into a thick bird's nest. The heat pushes proteins and synthetic polymers into the hair's shaft making it super-strong. The treatment lasts for months.

At home there are some excellent quick fixes. Hair, like skin, needs exfoliating because it collects chemicals, dust and product. Antonia suggests rinsing them out with **FREDERIC FEKKAI'S APPLE CIDER RINSE** or **KEVIN MURPHY'S MAXI WASH**, which contains AHAs to remove dead cells from the scalp and hair. Hair also ages just like skin. There's now a slew of anti-ageing hair-care lines, from **KERASTASE VITA-CIMENT** to **FREDERIC FEKKAI** and **CHARLES WORTHINGTON TIME DEFY**. I don't have the patience for sitting with a hair mask on for half an hour, but one of the best and quickest masks is **AVEDA'S COLOR CONSERVE STRENGTHENING TREATMENT**. Whack it on in the shower for five minutes and your hair will feel soft and silky.

the face

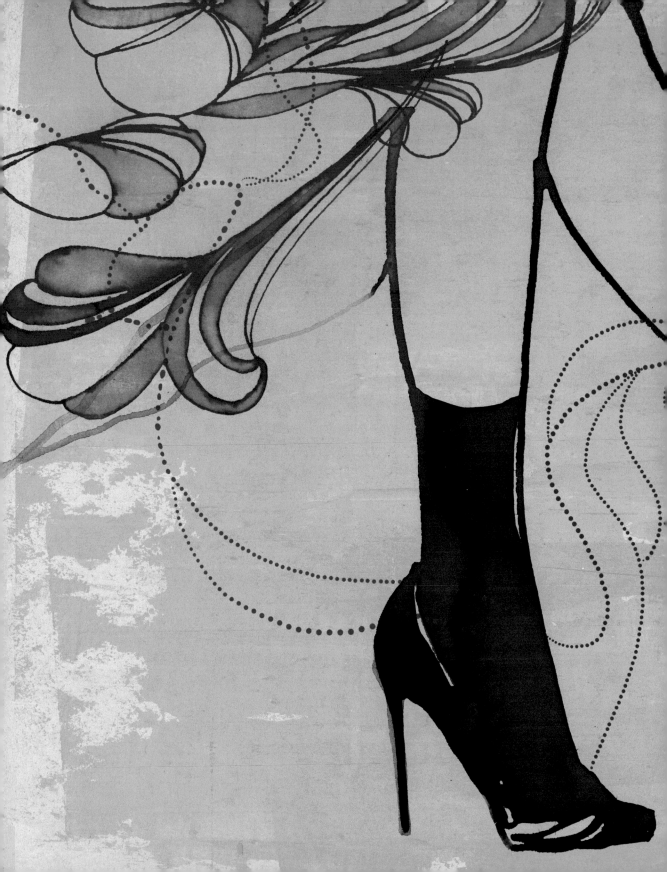

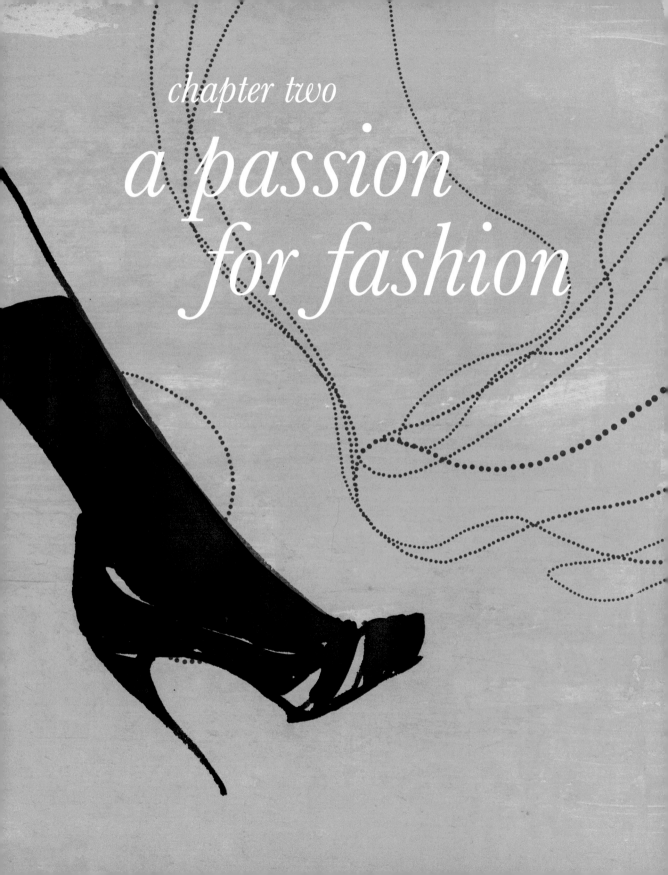

chapter two

a passion
for fashion

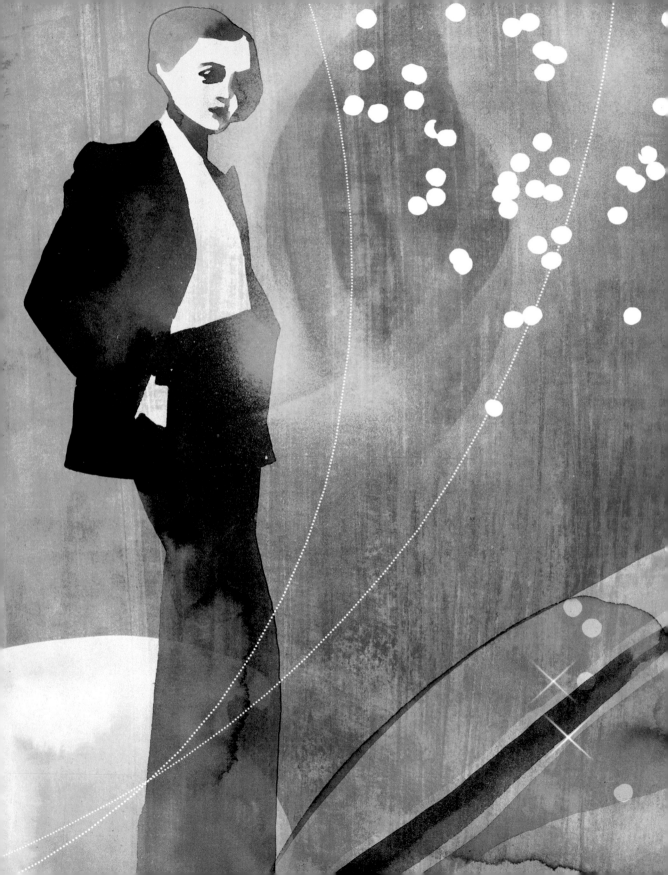

THE THINGS <u>WE DO</u> FOR FASHION!

THESE ARE JUST A FEW EXAMPLES OF WHAT WE'VE BEEN DOING TO OURSELVES FOR CENTURIES IN THE NAME OF FASHION, AND WHAT WE CONTINUE TO DO . . .

● **RECENT HISTORY MIGHT HAVE US BELIEVE BIKINIS WERE INVENTED IN THE FIFTIES.** How about 50 BC, or even earlier? Bikinis appear in wall paintings in Sri Lanka and in Minoan wall paintings dated 1600 BC.

● *HENRY VIII AND HIS MATES HAD A VERY SAUCY TIME. Women exposed their breasts, nipples and all. We think it's shocking on the catwalks today, but it's not new.*

● **QUEEN ELIZABETH I WAS FAMOUS FOR PUTTING A WHITE CHALK PASTE ON HER FACE** to look pale and interesting. Of course it ruined the skin and poisoned many of those who followed her example, as the paste was made from lead.

- *IN JANE AUSTEN'S DAY IT WASN'T UNKNOWN FOR WOMEN* to put on their dresses while they were still damp to ensure a body-clinging wet look, giving them a sexy image and pneumonia at the same time.

- **IN THE VICTORIAN ERA**, women suffered in corsets that squashed their organs and restricted the supply of oxygen to their lungs, hence they were forever fainting and needing smelling salts to revive them. Even more seriously, women often suffered from a prolapsed womb as the result of a brutal whalebone in the corsetry department.

- *THEY ALSO WORE BUM-ENLARGING BUSTLES. Do you think women asked each other, 'Does my bum look big enough in this?' I actually love bustles. Long skirts with bustles and corsets have been fun to wear on stage. They take a while to get used to but give you great posture. Also, you can't eat too much in a corset. Now there's an idea: the corset diet! Still, I'm happier in my jeans.*

● **WOMEN TORTURING THEMSELVES TO LOOK GOOD IS NOT A NEW THING**. Currently, we're debating the whole size-zero subject, which, when put into historical perspective, is a new variation on an old problem. And if you travelled east a hundred years ago, you'd have seen a much more drastic exercise in trying to achieve an attractive dainty foot than today's bunion-inducing stilettos. Mothers deliberately limited the growth of their daughters' feet from a young age, by binding them in tight bandages. This was thought to help make them more attractive to a prospective husband.

● *IN THE 1920S, WOMEN WOULD HAVE THEIR BREASTS BOUND TO FLATTEN THEM, so that they would fit into fashionable flapper dresses. During the Second World War, when women couldn't get hold of nylons for a dance, they would draw a black seam line from heel to bottom in pen and stain their legs with teabags. The first fake tan!*

● **GLOBALLY, THERE ARE STILL TRIBES THAT SEVER THE LOWER LIP** and insert a wooden plate so that they end up with a saucer-shaped mouth. Others have metal bands placed round their necks and add new ones each year, resulting in elongated necks. If the bands are removed, the muscles are so weak the head cannot be supported.

a passion for fashion

SHOE TIMELINE: *high heels*

2000 BC Greek horsemen and hunters wore 'cothurnus', a thick cork platform shoe

1500s Heels were introduced more widely for men to help prevent their feet from falling out of stirrups. So in fact they wore heels before the ladies

Mid 1500s Platforms and heels came into fashion, frequently fur-trimmed and bejewelled

1600s Venetian courtesans sported twenty-four-inch wedges to demonstrate their wealth and status

Mid 1600s Louis XIV heels were developed for the king; women began to sport 'Louis' heels

1745 Mme de Pompadour wore toe-constricting shoes with narrow heels and set a trend

1793 Marie Antoinette was executed wearing heels

Mid 1800s The plimsoll was invented for tennis

1950s A brand-new towering heel, known as the 'stiletto', was invented in Italy. Women never looked back

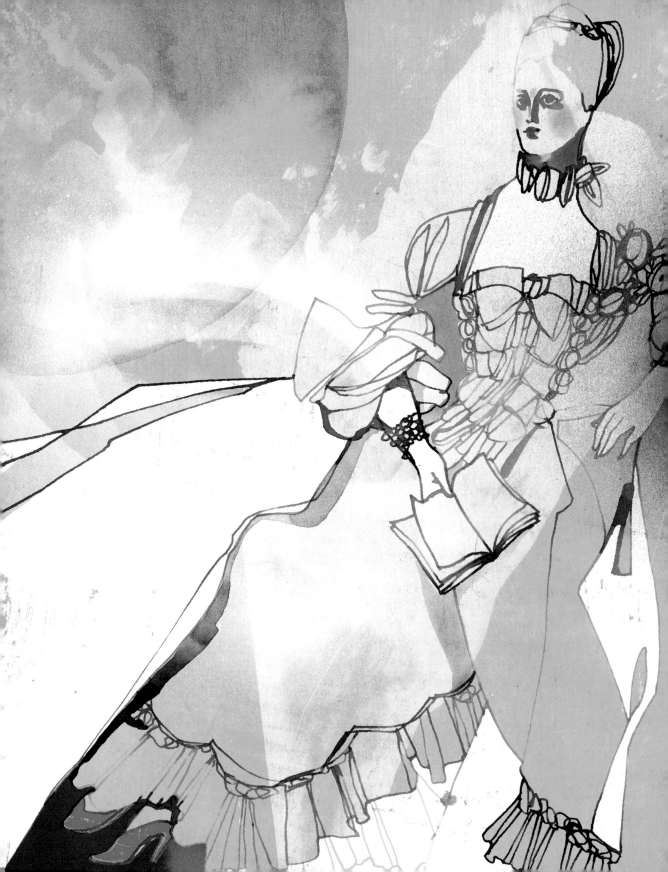

style icon

a passion for fashion

LOTS OF PEOPLE HAVE ASKED ME OVER THE YEARS WHO INSPIRES ME. WHEN IT COMES TO YOUR OWN PERSONAL STYLE, IT IS ALWAYS HELPFUL TO HAVE AN ICON IN MIND. IN OTHER WORDS, SOMEONE WHOSE STYLE YOU LOVE AND WISH TO EMULATE.

My favourite film stars were Greta Garbo and Merle Oberon, but your inspiration doesn't have to be a screen goddess, it could be one of your best friends. Mine was – and still is – Biba founder and genius designer, Barbara Hulanicki. When I first met Barbara in the late sixties, she completely took my breath away. I'd never seen such a stylish woman. She was the first designer to bring affordable, fashionable clothing to teenagers and was more responsible than anyone else for the popularity of the miniskirt. She was also always one step ahead of the pack. While we were all still busy sporting our minis, she created the antithesis to that look with wonderful, romantic wrap-around jersey dresses with big skirts, art deco prints and 1930s shapes. They were amazing. She used to send me, by taxi, packages of Biba dresses in every colour. Lucky me. In the same way that I looked different from anyone else when I first hit the fashion scene, so did she. I'd wear her clothes religiously. She is still one of my great friends. I learned such a lot about style, clothes and fabric from her. I knew how to sew from an early age, but Barbara was my biggest inspiration and always has been. As she has grown older, Barbara has kept her signature overall look, but she still looks stylish and modern.

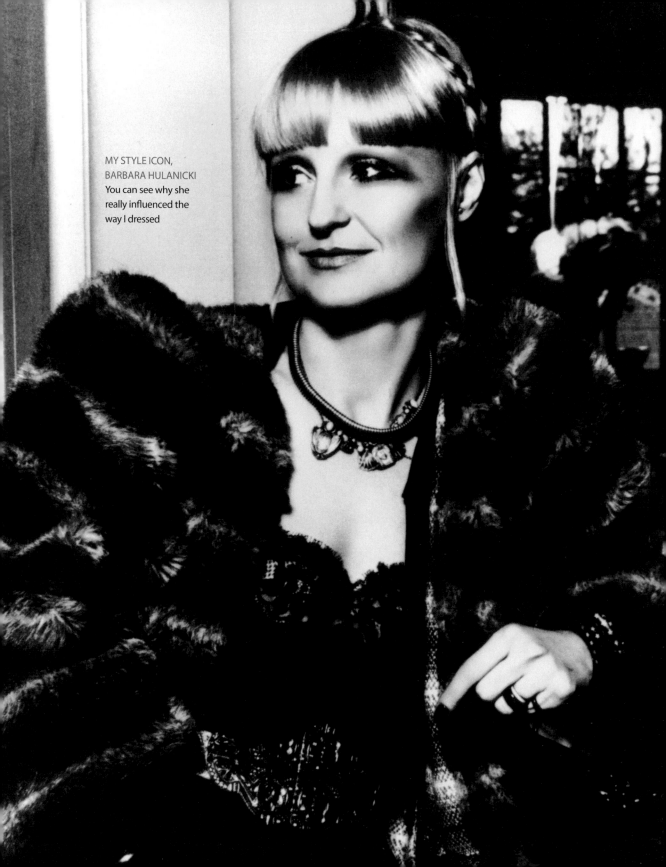

MY STYLE ICON,
BARBARA HULANICKI
You can see why she
really influenced the
way I dressed

colouring in

BLACK IS THE NEW BLACK

DARK COLOURS, BUT ESPECIALLY BLACK, CAN HELP YOUR LUMPS AND BUMPS DISAPPEAR. Black also makes you feel safe. Why do you think black is so favoured by the fashion pack? It's the ultimate uniform colour. When in doubt, many of my friends opt for black. It is a serious colour, great for business. One of my friends often dresses head to toe in black, yet, despite being a mother of three and a high-powered business woman, she isn't shy of a killer heel for work – Christian Louboutin platform mules, to be precise! Her hair and make-up are always impeccable, and her personality is strong and sexy enough to carry it off. I have another friend in LA who only wears black. It makes getting dressed a cinch, she says. Another friend buys only white, black and navy as it makes her wardrobe much simpler. Find your way of dressing, as it says so much about who you are. Black velvet is fabulous for evening; black T-shirts are perfect for wearing underneath a tailored jacket; black trousers are flattering on any shape or size. That's not to say my wardrobe is completely awash with black. I love bright colours too.

a passion for fashion

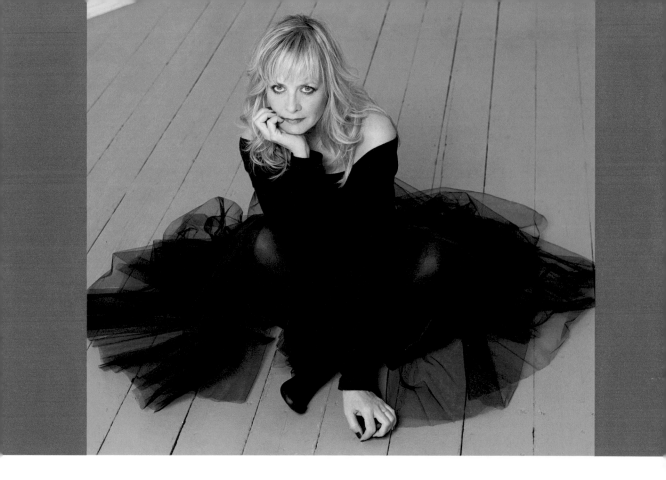

How to choose the right colour for you

This is a great tip suggested by fashion designer Betty Jackson: when you are thinking of trying a new colour, hold the garment right beside your face and compare it against the colour of your eyes and your overall skin tone. This makes it much easier to tell if it clashes with your colouring or enhances it. As with make-up, this kind of test is best done in daylight.

If you have high colouring, it is best to avoid bright red, but if you adore the colour, why not go for a pair of red shoes or an accessory in your favourite bright colour instead? If I'm going for colour I love purple, navy, brown, dark green, burgundy, anything but pale pink, pale blue, lime green or yellow – not good for blondes! Navy and grey are other friends to have in the wardrobe. Not quite as harsh as black, they mix so well with other colours. Lots of women get stuck in a rut with colours. We all feel safe with black and navy, but let's not forget bright colours too.

PRINTS CHARMING

I'M NOT A PRINT GIRL, PERSONALLY, AND HAVE ALWAYS FOUND THEM QUITE TRICKY. My daughter Carly, who is on the design team at Stella McCartney, is obsessed with them. I love the early Biba textiles, Liberty and Celia Birtwell prints, as well as the prints created during the 1930s. These are always soft and lovely. But as for swirls and big patterns, forget it! A small, subtle pattern can work brilliantly, I have very few patterned pieces in my wardrobe. If I'm wearing jeans I might wear a patterned top in muted hues.

Dress in patterns from head to toe and you're likely to fall foul of someone asking you if you're wearing the curtains! There can be a tendency to see the print and not the person. Choose summery print dresses carefully. Too loud and they may swamp you. If you still love a print, go for a top or skirt rather than head to toe.

I think wearing a bold print usually gets harder as you get older. It's safer to stick to subtle prints or block colours

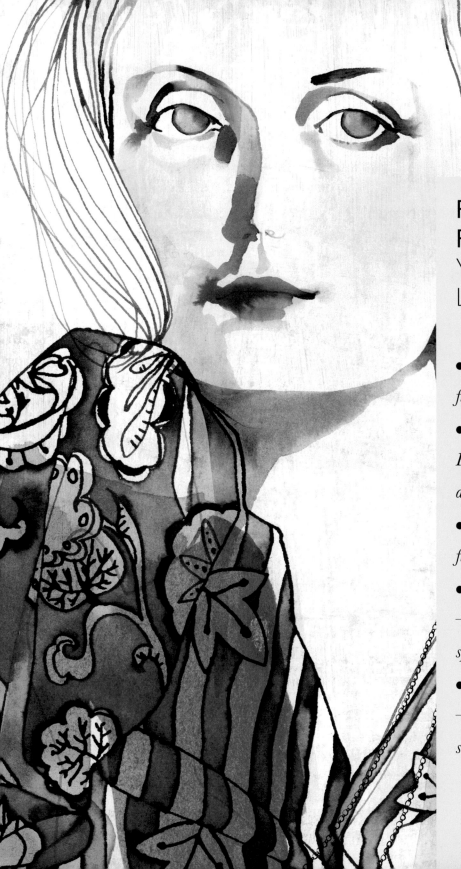

FOR GREAT FLORALS
YOU MIGHT LIKE TO TRY

- *HOBBS – classic floral silk dresses*
- *JIGSAW – English-rose print dresses and blouses*
- *KEW – good for floral-print separates*
- *LAURA ASHLEY – great for cotton-print spring tops and dresses*
- *L.K. BENNETT – look for their signature floral dresses*

STRIPES

STRIPES CAN BE TRICKY TOO. IF YOU'RE LARGER THAN A TWELVE, HORIZONTAL STRIPES ARE BEST AVOIDED. For small-breasted women, stripes can be fabulous as the curves of the body don't interrupt the stripe. A friend of mine is addicted to stripes. She has worn them ever since the age of four and has no intention of giving them up. Even when she was breastfeeding her kids with enormous boobs, the stripy Breton fisherman tops were worn with pride. Vertical stripes in trousers can be very flattering and sometimes, it's okay to break the rules . . .

VELVET

I LOVE VELVET. WHATEVER YOUR BODY SHAPE AND SIZE, VELVET IS SO SUMPTUOUS AND BEAUTIFUL. It is also a lovely fabric to wear at Christmas. I have a gorgeous crushed-velvet evening coat by Ghost, which has lasted years. There's nothing like velvet for a posh frock; it's a chic option for smart trousers too. A velvet blazer with jeans is a fabulous look for day.

FOR STRIPES YOU MIGHT LIKE TO TRY

- *A.P.C. – for classic French easy-chic tops*
- *BODEN – always do cotton striped tops in various colours*
- *JOULES – classic British easy-weekend styles*
- *THE ORIGINAL BRETON SHIRT COMPANY – offers different colours plus the classic blue and white Breton*

I made this velvet dress myself, from beautiful fabric I bought in Italy

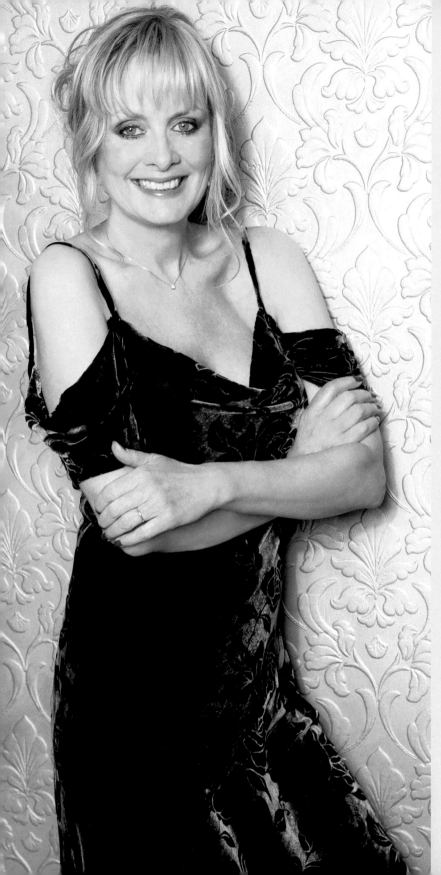

FOR VELVET JACKETS, COATS AND DRESSES YOU MIGHT LIKE TO TRY

- *Liberty*
- *Jaeger*
- *Joseph*
- *Diane Von Furstenberg*

FOR SCARVES AND WRAPS YOU MIGHT LIKE TO TRY

- *Georgina Von Etzdorf*
- *Charles & Patricia Lester*
- *M&S*
- *Tie Rack*

wardrobe
maintenance

THE SIN BIN

WE ALL HAVE FASHION NO-NOS LURKING IN OUR WARDROBES.

WHAT TO BIN

- SLOGAN T-SHIRTS
- THONGS. There's nothing dignified about these and they are so uncomfortable!
- CULOTTES. I've always hated them! How can anyone look good in them? If you're thin, you end up looking like Weed from *Bill and Ben*, or it looks like your trousers have shrunk. If you're plump, they just make you look short. Every pair should be burned
- CROPPED TOPS. Certainly not for us fortysomethings – don't even go there
- HIPSTER JEANS WORN TO REVEAL YOUR TUMMY. If you do love them, team them with big sweaters or shirts
- You don't want to go and buy the boring old CREAM MACKINTOSH or the PASTEL SHORTIE ANORAKS either!
- TOO-TIGHT TROUSERS. If they are too small round the waist they bunch up around the button and cause a floppy overspill
- PALE BLUE AND PALE GREEN EYESHADOW
- BABY-PINK LIPSTICK. Brigitte Bardot? Don't fool yourself!
- WHITE SKIN-TIGHT TROUSERS. Especially ones with polyester!
- THIN DENIER TIGHTS

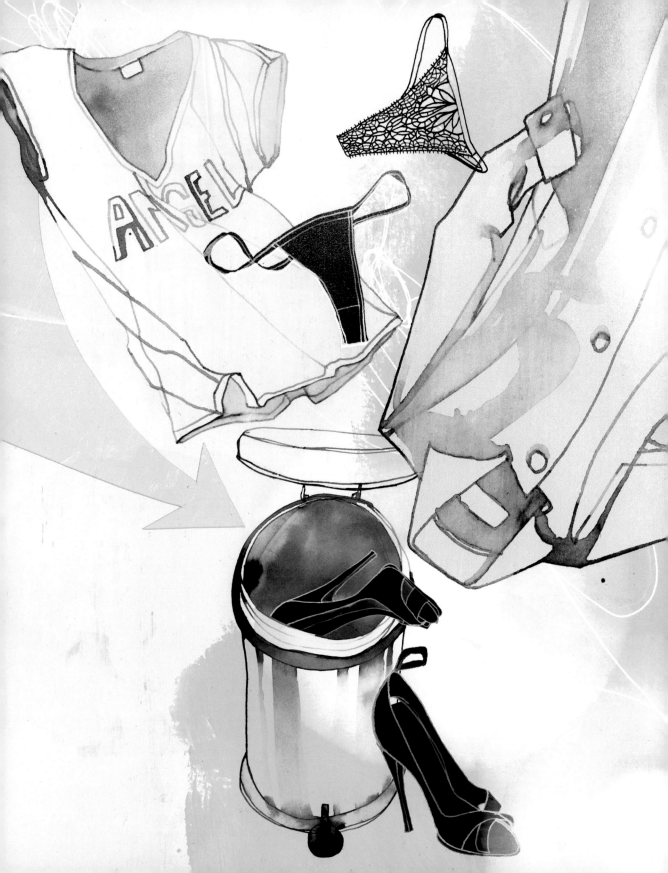

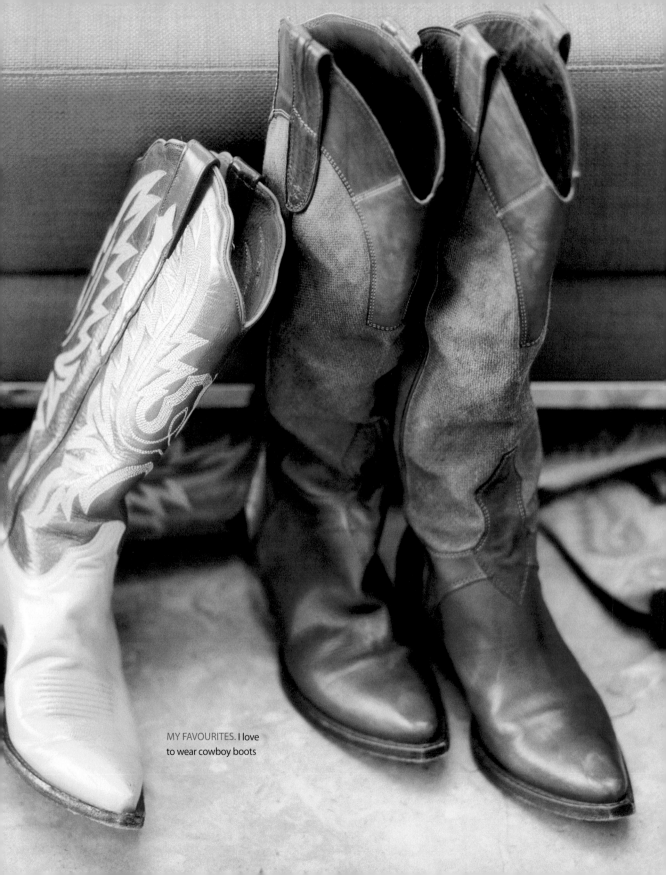

MY FAVOURITES. I love
to wear cowboy boots

- **SHOES YOU CAN'T WALK IN.** Mind you, I've got loads of those too . . . they're lovely to look at!
- **HALTER-NECK TOPS** in very large sizes
- **I CAN'T WEAR YELLOW**, but if you're very dark it looks wonderful
- Trousers that give you a camel's hoof. **BEWARE THE TIGHT CROTCH ZONE!**
- **VPL-ERS.** These must only be worn with loose garments. Basic cotton, high-leg briefs are lovely and comfy if I'm not wearing anything figure-hugging
- Unless it's for a special occasion at home with a special person, **AVOID FRILLY UNDERWEAR**

WHAT TO KEEP

There's no use having gorgeous clothes if they are not looked after and stored properly. When we bought our flat in London, I never had enough room for my clothes. Eventually, I stole the spare bedroom and converted it into a walk-in wardrobe/dressing room. Despite this extravagant use of space, I still need more room! You don't need a palatial walk-in wardrobe to achieve a well-organized wardrobe system. Truth is, the bigger the wardrobe, the more likely you are to fill it to the brim.

Here's how I arrange my wardrobe

- **HIGH RAILS** to avoid folding over for skirts, long dresses and trousers. Another high rail for long jackets, frock coats and coats
- **A LOW RAIL** for jackets and waistcoats
- **BIG CUBICLE CUPBOARDS** with shelves for: leggings, tracksuits, scarves, sarongs. Plus other shelves for undies, socks and vests
- **SHOES** are all stored along the bottom of the shelves on the floor, not in boxes, but placed in pairs for easy access
- I've also got endless **BOOTS** and I'll never throw any away. I love boots more than anything. I think it's a disease – bootitus!
- **HATS AND SUITCASES** are stored on top of the wardrobes

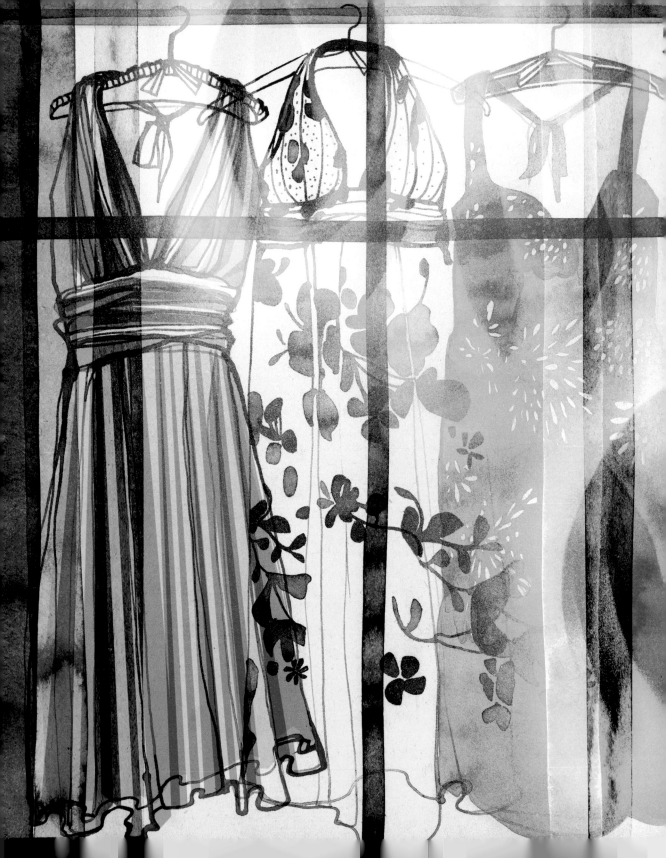

It's no bad thing to have a sort-out once or twice a year. Doing so is very cathartic, as long as you are recycling properly. Never, ever throw stuff out! Instead, recycle everything. In my house, it goes to family, friends of family and charity shops. It's not necessary to buy a new wardrobe every season. I've got lots of things in my wardrobe I have had for years and worn and worn. Leigh bought me a coat in 1988 and I still wear it and love it. Made of thick fleece with purple piping, it's the ultimate coat for a cold day. It's also fabulous for travelling and I can bung it in the wash.

Don't be pressured into following the 'throw everything out that hasn't been worn in over a year' rule. It's total rubbish. Obviously, if clothes don't fit you any more it's worth reassessing the value of holding on to them, but favourite pieces can serve as an incentive to eat a bit more sensibly, exercise more and shed a few pounds. If you love an outfit, keep it long enough and it will come back into fashion. Like so many of my girlfriends, I go through phases of wearing something over and over, then getting bored of it, hiding it away, and then a few years later coming across it . . . and the cycle repeats.

Look after your precious dresses by hanging them on padded hangers. Wire hangers will destroy the shoulders on silk dresses if left in the wardrobe year after year

I have tons of old favourites from over the years that I know I'll bring out every few years and wear with something else, or reinvent by teaming with a recent purchase

Keep sweaters folded and keep lavender, cedar and sandalwood in the wardrobe to repel moths. I'm probably the only person in the world who loves the smell of mothballs. Don't ask me why, but to the majority of people mothballs smell dreadful. Be ruthless if you spot a moth. Clear everything out, put your cashmere in the freezer for twenty-four hours to get rid of infestation, hoover every nook and cranny and dry-clean all precious items. If you have a really bad infestation, you can get professionals in to spray the house.

If, like me, you have a few favourite holiday pieces, it's a good idea to fold them away with your swimsuits and sunhats. It makes packing for holidays so much easier when the time comes. Holiday clothes don't ever go out of fashion. That's why I have a stash of favourites such as cotton gypsy skirts, sundresses, kaftans and sarongs, collected over the years.

If you are short on space, vacuum bags are a lifesaver. They can shrink four sweaters down to the size of an A4 envelope! The best ones I have found are the **STACK AND VAC BAGS** from **LAKELAND** (every homeowner's guilty pleasure). It's great to use these bags for storing away bulky wintry items in high summer, and vice versa.

WARDROBE STAPLES

THERE ARE CERTAIN ITEMS WORTH KEEPING ALL YEAR ROUND

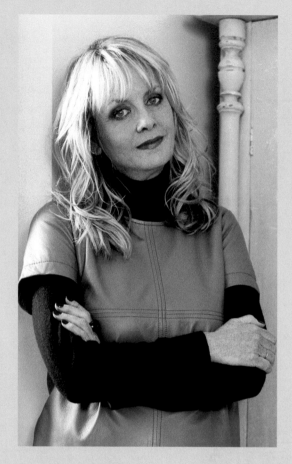

- **BLACK POLO-NECK SWEATERS** in varying thicknesses, from cashmere to knitted cottons. For me, they're a great basic for wearing under a trouser suit, with a skirt and under a bigger jumper for warmth in the winter. The following are great places to investigate for this wardrobe staple: N. PEAL, BRORA, M&S, UNIQLO, GAP, KEW, DEBENHAMS, BHS, H&M. The only time to steer clear of polo necks is if you have a short neck. Otherwise, they flatter everyone and are great for coverage too.

- **LOW V-NECK, LONG-SLEEVED SWEATERS** – I also love to wear these very clingy, in various thicknesses – warm cashmeres, knitted cotton, fine/sheer knit jersey. They are brilliant for wearing underneath sleeveless tops as well as on their own. A slinky one with a full skirt, a pencil skirt or a pair of tight jeans and a big belt looks great. It works brilliantly as an evening outfit too, with a giant skirt and necklace.

- **JEANS.** They are seasonless.

- **BOOTS.** These I wear more than shoes, even in summer. A summer dress with soft boots looks fabulous if you have brown legs. If you don't, get out the fake tan!

packing

WHAT TO PACK IS A CONUNDRUM. I ALWAYS TAKE WAY TOO MUCH WITH ME AND END UP WEARING ONLY A THIRD OF WHAT I HAVE PACKED. Some of my friends are whizzes at packing the right amount of clothing for a holiday. One of my friends rolls everything up before putting it in a suitcase, and that certainly helps on space. Another friend lays out everything that she wants to take with her on her bed, then ruthlessly halves it. I tried that for a trip to South Africa recently and it worked a treat!

If you are going somewhere hot, however much you pack it's handy to have a mini collection of summery kaftans, skirts and dresses, as these can be lifesavers not only for coverage when you're not actually swimming in the sea or pool, or sunbathing, but they are also the most comfortable things to wear in the heat.

I also swear by a couple of different-sized sarongs. One is just enough to cover the hips and bum, which I love pre-swim, the other is the size of a single bed sheet. You can use it as something comfy to lie on and it doubles up as a modesty curtain when you've had a swim and want to get out of your wet bathing suit. Simply hold it around yourself like a giant bath towel, cross both corners over and tie them at the neck. Voila! You can remove your swimsuit and you have a chic robe.

For evening, there's nothing simpler than a scrunchy silk skirt with an elasticated waist. These are so easy to pack as they reduce to a tiny ball. Best of all, they don't require any ironing. Hooray! I'll bung one on with a vest top, pretty blouse and belt. I don't bother taking heels on holiday as there're usually cobbled stone streets, so I tend to wear sandals. I always pack a pair of trainers as back-up and for rocky walks. For evenings, flip-flops can be dressy. Holidays are the only time I'll ever wear shorts. Unless you're under twenty-four or in the back garden, I would advise you not to wear short shorts. Loose Indian cotton tops are lovely for holidays, as are very soft cotton or linen drawstring trousers. I also love fatigue trousers in bright colours. Loose-fitting clothes are so much comfier if you're catching the sun. There's nothing worse than scorched skin in tight clothes.

KAFTANS

WHETHER YOU ARE GOING TO THE BEACH for a long weekend or for a fortnight, consider the three-kaftan rule:

1 **KAFTAN ONE:** for covering the bum and throwing on after swims – or before, with your bathing suit underneath.

2 **KAFTAN TWO:** down to the knee, enough coverage to have lunch in, with bathing suit underneath; also looks great with floaty linen trousers or jeans.

3 **KAFTAN THREE:** ankle-length, perfect for après sun or for wearing in the evening with a nice pair of sparkly flat sandals.

KAFTANS YOU MIGHT LIKE TO TRY

- *ACCESSORIZE – affordable and perfect for last-minute getaways*

- *ALLEGRA HICKS – for a designer A-list kaftan, these are sublime*

- *ANYA HINDMARCH – effortlessly stylish and a great investment*

- *HEIDI KLEIN – luxurious, sexy and available all year round*

- *LIZA BRUCE – beautifully crafted in silk chiffon and sequins*

- *M&S – amazing, exotic, animal-print chiffon kaftans*

- *WALLIS – great beach cover-ups in subtle colours*

BIKINIS

I COLLECT BIKINIS. I LOVE THEM! Bikini tops with Grecian gathering are flattering on any shape. I like getting my tummy brown. There are no rules about when to stop wearing bikinis. If you feel confident about it, wear a bikini at any age! You can always wear a sarong for coverage. I personally don't think there's any point in spending too much on a bikini as the chlorine and sea water tend to shorten their shelf life anyway. At least, that's my excuse . . .

WEEKENDS AWAY

HERE'S A HANDY HINT FOR PACKING FOR A WEEKEND/CITY BREAK. Imagine you are only allowed ten items. What would they be?

Here are mine
1. PAIR OF SKINNY (NOT ESSENTIAL) JEANS (ESSENTIAL), PROBABLY BLACK
2. PAIR OF SCRUNCHY, COMFY BOOTS
3. PAIR OF BALLET PUMPS
4. BLACK SWEATER
5. TAILORED JACKET
6. KNEE-LENGTH SKIRT
7. WHITE SHIRT
8. BRIGHTLY COLOURED PASHMINA
9. TOP THAT COULD WORK OFF THE SHOULDER FOR EVENING
10. SHORT STRING OF PEARLS

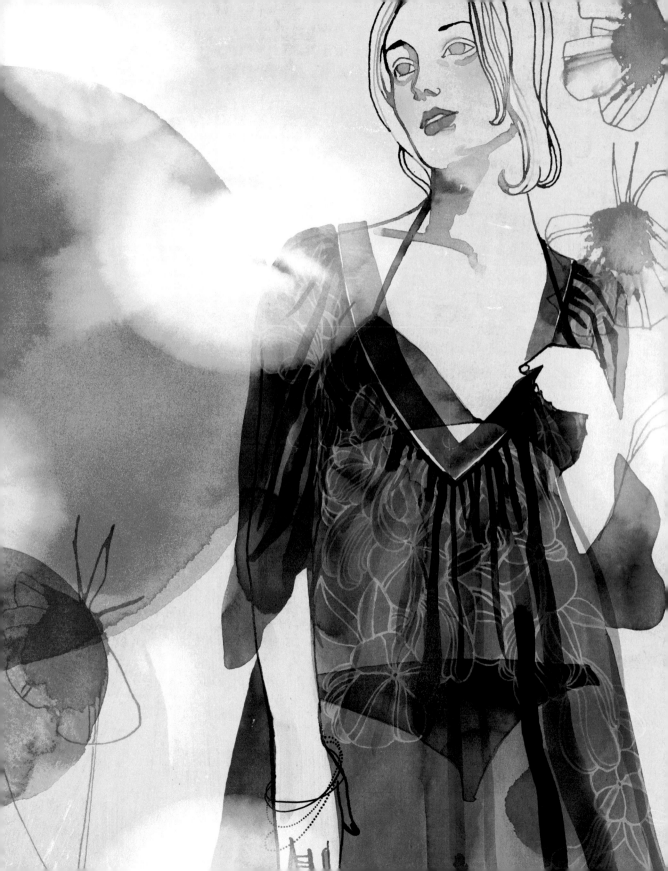

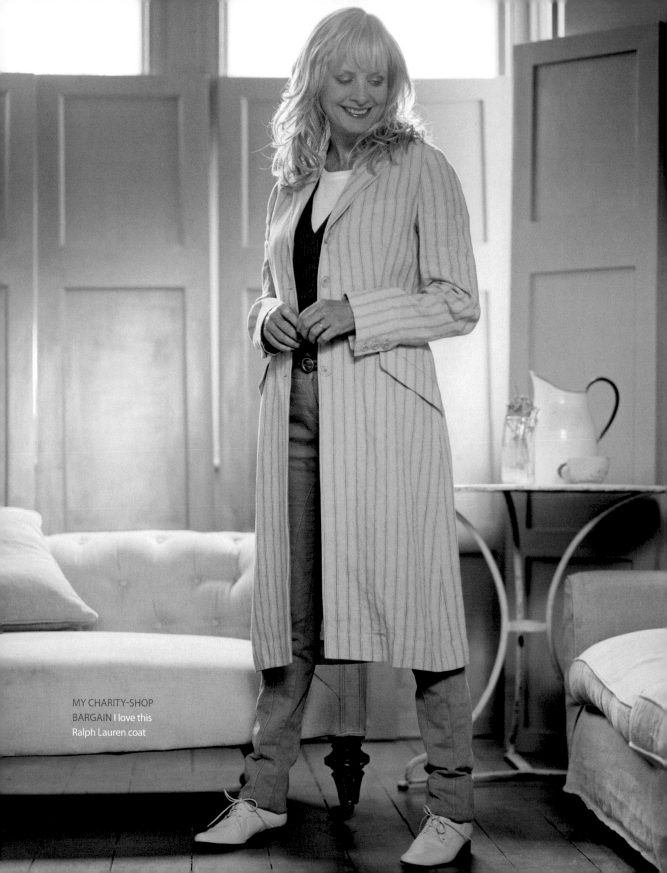

MY CHARITY-SHOP
BARGAIN I love this
Ralph Lauren coat

shopping

I DON'T KNOW ABOUT YOU BUT I LOVE SHOPPING. BEFORE YOU EMBARK ON A SHOPPING SPREE, BE IN THE RIGHT MOOD. PANIC BUYING IS ALWAYS GOING TO END UP IN A CRISIS. If you're feeling insecure or unsure about what to choose, look around at your friends and ask the one whose style you love best to help you. Make sure she is the kind of friend who can be objective and will listen to your insecurities rather than allow her own style agenda to take over. Be honest with your shopping partner-in-crime. Tell her you need objectivity from her. Shop together and try stuff on without feeling obliged to buy. If you feel there's something missing in your wardrobe, set aside a bit of time and have some fun experimenting with different silhouettes. Go to a few shops you've never visited before and don't be put off by the youthful marketing. You'll be pleasantly surprised by the choices there for you, so long as you take the plunge and go for it. Although helpful, it's not enough to believe what the shop assistant says. After all, it's her job to get you to buy something! Learn to trust your instinct. Go with what feels right. If you are unsure, put it on hold and take a friend back with you for a second opinion before buying.

Sometimes the best personal shopper can be your daughter. Carly and I shop together a lot and we're both really honest with each other. I can always count on her to say, 'Muuuuuuuuuuuum!' if she thinks I'm making a rotten choice, and vice versa.

125

LABELS

WHICH DO YOU PREFER, DESIGNER OR HIGH STREET? I know women who will only buy posh labels. It's a personal choice, of course. If you've got lots of dosh you can go down that route and invest in beautiful things that last and last. But if you can't afford to do that, there is no reason not to be stylish and fashionable and keep in budget. You might assume I only wear designer labels, but to tell you the truth I absolutely love high-street clothes.

What I'm trying to say is that, whatever your budget, it is still possible to find terrific clothes. So much of the high street may seem to be targeting teenagers and young 'uns, but I know plenty of girls my age, and some of them are grannies, who buy bits and pieces from these stores and look great. The trick is to know what suits you. Once you have established that, you can shop anywhere!

BARGAIN SHOPPING

MY FRIENDS KNOW ME AS THE BARGAIN SHOPPER OF THE WORLD. If I see a big sale sign going up I go in and somehow manage to find wonderful things. It's such a thrill when you can snap up a discount bargain; it's good for the soul as well as the pocket. Designer sample sales are a great opportunity to splurge on pieces that might otherwise feel too extravagant. Mind you, you're just as likely to find me scouring the charity-shop rails. At Oxfam recently, I was flipping through the hangers and found the most beautiful cream-linen man's frock coat by Ralph Lauren *(see p.124)*, perfect condition, in my size, for £25. I was over the moon!

One of my favourite jackets in the world was bought from a garage sale in LA. There was a guy with a rail of 1940s pieces. I picked up this Prince of Wales checked jacket with slanted buttonholes and a Peter Pan collar. Price? $20. I wear it so often. I love charity shops and vintage.

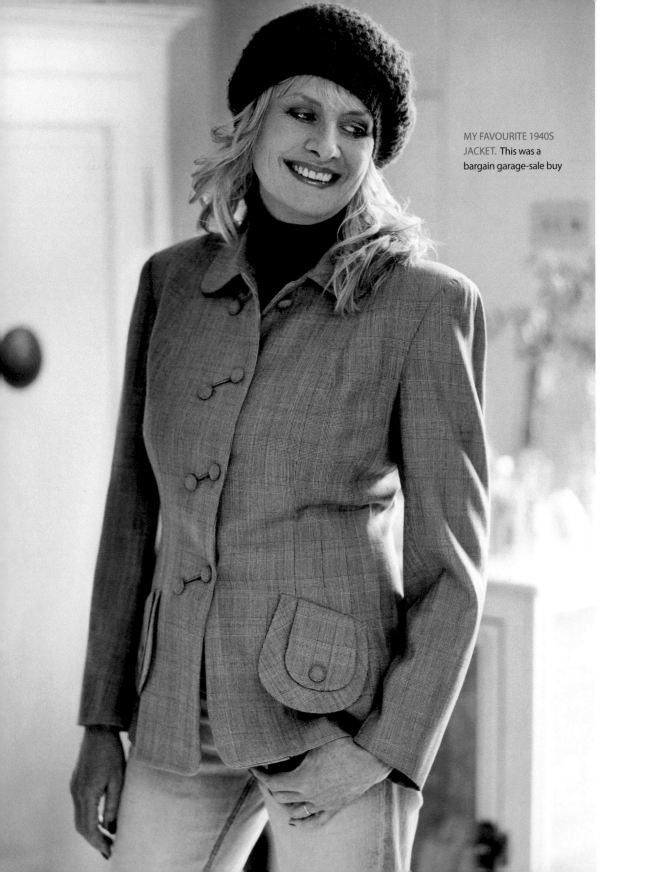

MY FAVOURITE 1940S
JACKET. This was a
bargain garage-sale buy

Don't think of charity shops or vintage as second-hand, think of it as the ultimate in recycling chic!

The best charity shops are in the posh neighbourhoods as a lot of wealthy women donate unworn designer gear to their local store. Second-hand designer clothes stores are also a great way to invest in a special jacket, dress or shirt without breaking the bank.

Think of charity shopping as doing your bit for the environment! Also check your local newspaper for antique clothes fairs.

TOP TIPS

IF YOU SEE SOMETHING YOU REALLY, REALLY LOVE, DON'T BUY IT ON THE SPOT. Try it on, ask the store to hold it for a day or a few days. Go away and think about it. If you keep going back to it, chances are it's a good choice.

One woman who knows a lot about style is Joan Burstein CBE, the elegant owner and founder of Browns in South Molton Street, in London. Mrs B, as she is affectionately known, has worked in the fashion industry for sixty years, much of that time as a buyer. Now in her eighties, she is a seasoned expert on how to make your wardrobe your best friend.

Here are <u>Mrs B's</u> tips

1 **FIND A SHOP YOU LIKE** with a sales assistant who understands your needs and keeps you informed when new things come in that would suit you.

2 **GO FOR QUALITY IN FABRICS AND TAILORING.** These will be a better investment in the long run as they will last.

3 **PAY ATTENTION TO ACCESSORIES,** as they can completely change the mood of how you look. A nice scarf or piece of jewellery can make an outfit. And a good belt can easily restyle a dress.

4 **STICK TO ONE COLOUR**, or a limited colour palette. Notice how elegant the Queen looks when she dresses in one shade.

5 **LAYERING CAN BE EFFECTIVE** but must be done very carefully to avoid adding bulk to the problem areas of the body, i.e. the tummy and the hips. When layering tops, aim to cut the body off at the narrowest points, so as to create the illusion of a slimmer figure. A line across the tummy distracts the eye, whereas a top ending on the hips lengthens the body.

6 **DON'T BUY ITEMS THAT LOOK CHEAP** or poorly constructed, as they will do you no favours.

7 **GOOD GROOMING IS ESSENTIAL.** It is best to start with the hair and make-up, and the rest of the outfit will follow.

Some great stores to _shop_ at nationwide

1 LONDON BOUTIQUES

- **ANNA** – Good mid-range prices and great labels for forty-plus women (Anna is one of the most stylish forty-plus women you'll ever meet!)

- **BROWNS** – stocks classic and avant-garde designers, from **BALENCIAGA** to JIL SANDER

- **FEATHERS** – contains a fabulous selection of European designers including **ANN DEMEULEMEESTER** and **ALEXANDER MCQUEEN**

- **A LA MODE** – one of London's chicest boutiques, stocking the best of the best with bespoke service to match

- **MATCHES** – vibrant and stylish chain of boutiques, including a great selection of **CHLOÉ** and **LANVIN**, with excellent accessories

- **JOSEPH** – stocks a great range of labels including **PRADA** and **DOLCE & GABBANA**

2 REGIONAL BOUTIQUES

- ABERDEEN – **ZOOMP** – a vibrant store specializing in glamorous eveningwear by **BEN DE LISI**, **DOLCE & GABBANA** and **JUST CAVALLI** as well as quirky separates by **SONIA BY SONIA RYKIEL**.

- ASHBOURNE – **YOUNG IDEAS** – a stylish boutique gathering collections from **DONNA KARAN**, **DIANE VON FURSTENBERG**, **DRIES VAN NOTEN** and **PAUL SMITH** to more casual essentials from **C&C CALIFORNIA** and **SEVEN FOR ALL MANKIND** jeans.

- BARNSLEY – **POLLYANNA** – an über-chic and style-conscious institution in

a passion for fashion

130

the north. Pollyanna is known for stocking only the best from avant-garde designers, **COMME DES GARÇONS, JUNYA WATANABE, LANVIN** and **YVES SAINT LAURENT**.

- BATH – <u>**SQUARE**</u> – a quaint but very fashion-savvy clothes shop, stocking **MISSONI, MATTHEW WILLIAMSON** and evening dresses by **TEMPERLEY**. It also houses an amazing accessories store with a great range of **MARC JACOBS, PRADA** and **MIU MIU** shoes.

- BIRMINGHAM – <u>**SELFRIDGES**</u> – Set in the Bullring, this landmark is less of a boutique than a department store, but is a great place to pick up hot designer finds from **MARNI, MISSONI** and **SEE BY CHLOÉ** and boasts an excellent array of accessories from **MARC BY MARC JACOBS** to **CHLOÉ** and **VIVIENNE WESTWOOD**.

- BOURNEMOUTH – <u>**L'AMICA**</u> – a pretty boutique that caters for the professional woman who likes to dress well with a feminine edge, stocking **PAUL SMITH, PHILOSOPHY DI ALBERTA FERRETTI** and **DIANE VON FURSTENBERG**.

- CAMBRIDGE – <u>**GIULIO**</u> – houses an impressive array of **CHLOÉ, GUCCI** and **PRADA** clothes and accessories, located in Cambridge city centre.

- CARDIFF – <u>**BODY BASICS**</u> – stocks a good range of easily wearable classics from **BETTY JACKSON, MOSCHINO, DAY BIRGER ET MIKKELSEN, TOMMY HILFIGER** and **JOSEPH**. Prices are all very reasonable.

- CHESTER – <u>**TESSUTI**</u> – in the heart of Chester, houses both men's and women's fashions, with luxe labels

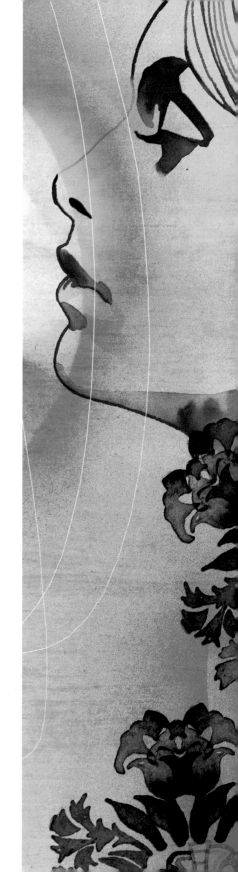

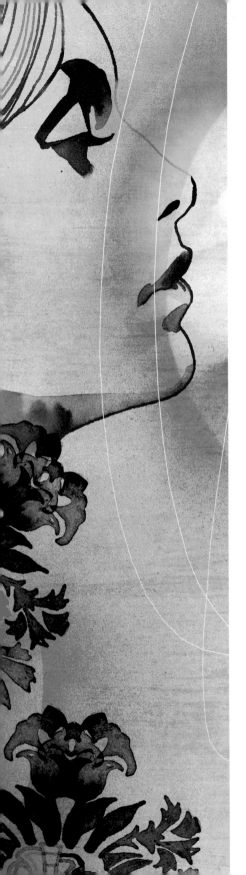

like **TEMPERLEY** and **MISSONI** sitting alongside cool **DVB** jeans, **MULBERRY** bags and **GINA** shoes.

- DUBLIN – <u>**BROWN THOMAS**</u> – this most elegant of designer department stores stocks the very best from top-end designers **GIANBATTISTA VALLI**, **MICHAEL KORS**, **DEREK LAM** and **DRIES VAN NOTEN**. Accessories have their own forum with must-have bags from **LUELLA**, **GUCCI**, **DOLCE & GABBANA** and **CHLOÉ**.

- EDINBURGH – <u>**JANE DAVIDSON**</u> – set in beautiful surroundings in a Georgian townhouse, Jane specializes in eveningwear by **JENNY PACKHAM** and **BEN DE LISI**, alongside beautiful separates from **PAUL & JOE** and slick denim from **ACNE** and **J BRAND**.

- ESHER – <u>**BERNARD OF ESHER**</u> – an institution in the rural south-east, this pretty boutique stocks a heady mix of romantic and ultra-feminine pieces by **STELLA MCCARTNEY**, **SEE BY CHLOÉ**, **MISSONI** and **VANESSA BRUNO**.

- GLASGOW – <u>**CRUISE**</u> – a high-end luxury men's and women's boutique that boasts a premium collection of women's clothes from **PAUL SMITH** to **HUGO BOSS** in addition to handbags by **VIVIENNE WESTWOOD** and **CHLOÉ** and **JIMMY CHOO** shoes.

- HARROGATE – <u>**THE CLOTHES ROOM**</u> – a local institution, just out of town, this store has a loyal clientele that flocks to buy **EDINA RONAY**, **NICOLE FARHI**, **BETTY JACKSON** and pretty dresses from **MEGAN PARK** and **ALLEGRA HICKS**.

- HUNGERFORD – **<u>JEANNE PETITT</u>** – a friendly and welcoming boutique that offers a mixture of designer casual pieces from **ANN LOUISE ROSWALD** and **EDINA RONAY** and beautiful eveningwear from **AMANDA WAKELEY**and **TEMPERLEY**.

- LIVERPOOL – **<u>CRICKET</u>** – a Liverpool institution, this little fashion shop has become ever popular amongst the WAGs and stocks an impressive range of glamorous dresses by **CHLOÉ**, **LANVIN** and **MATTHEW WILLIAMSON** as well as divine shoes by **MISSONI** and **BALENCIAGA**.

- MANCHESTER AND LEEDS – **<u>FLANNELS</u>** – a funky emporium of boutiques for fashion-savvy females, specializing in dressing-up frocks from **D&G**, **JUST CAVALLI** and **SONIA RYKIEL** and plenty of designer handbags from **FENDI** and **MARC BY MARC JACOBS**.

- NEWCASTLE – **<u>JULES B</u>** – an exciting treasure of a shop packed full of gorgeously feminine frocks from **DIANE VON FURSTENBERG**, **HOSS INTROPIA** and Sienna Miller's cool label, **TWENTY8TWELVE**.

- SOUTHAMPTON – **<u>REPERTOIRE</u>** – has a brilliant range of slick tailoring from **ARMANI** and **RALPH LAUREN** in addition to great separates from Joseph and piles of jeans from **J BRAND** to **ROCK & REPUBLIC**.

- ST ALBANS – **<u>RICHARD OLIVER</u>** – tucked away in St Albans, this treasure trove has both great eveningwear and workwear, from **PAUL SMITH** and **HUGO BOSS**.

- TORQUAY – **<u>MAGGIE & CO</u>** – top-end designer haven of posh frocks from **BEN DE LISI**, **AMANDA WAKELEY**, **DONNA KARAN** and **RALPH LAUREN**, plus gorgeous **MULBERRY** handbags.

- TRURO – **<u>BISHOP PHILPOTT</u>** – a fine boutique for the well-heeled south-west corner of England, great for workwear and tailoring from the likes of **PAUL SMITH**, **VIVIENNE WESTWOOD** and **NICOLE FARHI** as well as pretty dresses from **MEGAN PARK**.

- WINCHESTER – **<u>THE HAMBLEDON</u>** – a fantastically clean lifestyle store with gorgeous women's labels like **ANN LOUISE ROSWALD**, **MARGARET HOWELL**, **DAY BIRGER ET MIKKELSON** and **J&M DAVIDSON** sitting alongside beautiful homewares.

a passion for fashion

3 *BIG-NAME DEPARTMENT STORES*

Major department stores are a great place to one-stop shop. Generally they have a good range of reliable classics, workwear suits, great shoes, handbags, scarves and accessories. They're also invaluable for picking up extra pairs of tights, gloves and a woolly hat for when the weather turns cold and generally having everything under one roof. **HOUSE OF FRASER, DEBENHAMS, FENWICK** and **JOHN LEWIS** are all fabulous institutions, whilst **HARVEY NICHOLS** and **SELFRIDGES** now have stores in both the north and south of the country offering a great designer mecca. (*See list of general department stores on stockists pages.*)

4 *GREAT HIGH–STREET STORES*

We all love a bargain and the British high street has so much to offer. It's definitely worth shopping around, if you have the time. You may be surprised by what you find if you try out stores like **ALL SAINTS, ZARA, REISS, H&M** and **TOPSHOP** alongside more established brands like **GAP, JIGSAW, PRINCIPLES** and **HOBBS**. Shopping should be a pleasurable experience and the wealth of garments, trends, accessories and ideas out there are all waiting to be experienced. The beauty of the high street is that you don't have to spend a fortune, so try shopping outside your comfort zone . (*See list of high-street stores on stockists pages.*)

5 *GREAT HIGH-END DESIGNER STORES/BRANDS FOR CLASSIC DAY, EVENING AND WORKWEAR*

- ALBERTA FERRETTI ● BETTY JACKSON ● BRION ● BURBERRY ● CELINE ● CHANEL
- DKNY ● DOLCE & GABBANA ● DONNA KARAN ● GIORGIO & EMPORIO ARMANI
- J&M DAVIDSON ● JAEGER ● JOSEPH ● LOUIS VUITTON ● MARNI ● MATTHEW WILLIAMSON ● MAXMARA ● MOSCHINO ● PRADA ● RALPH LAUREN ● STELLA MCCARTNEY ● VIVIENNE WESTWOOD

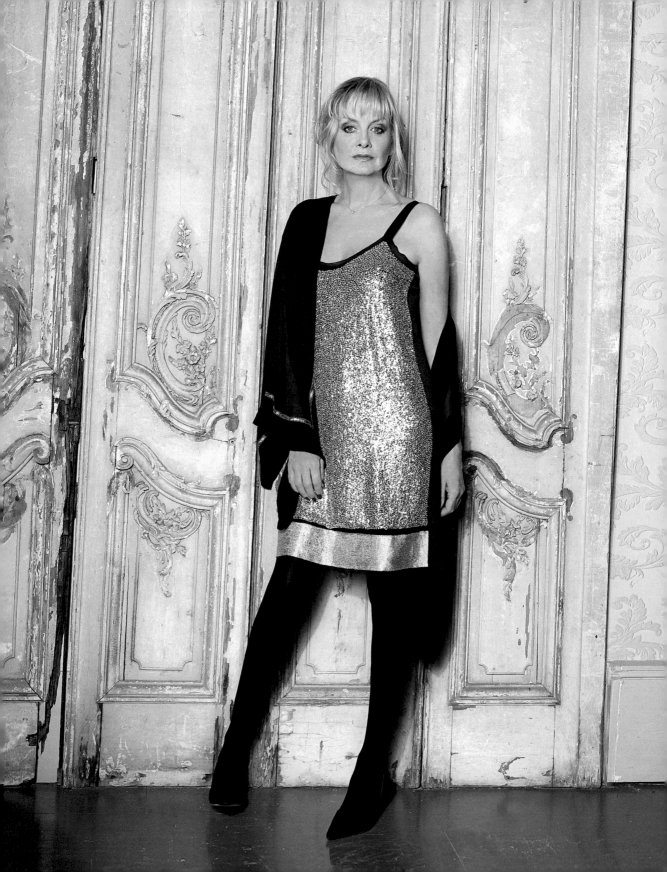

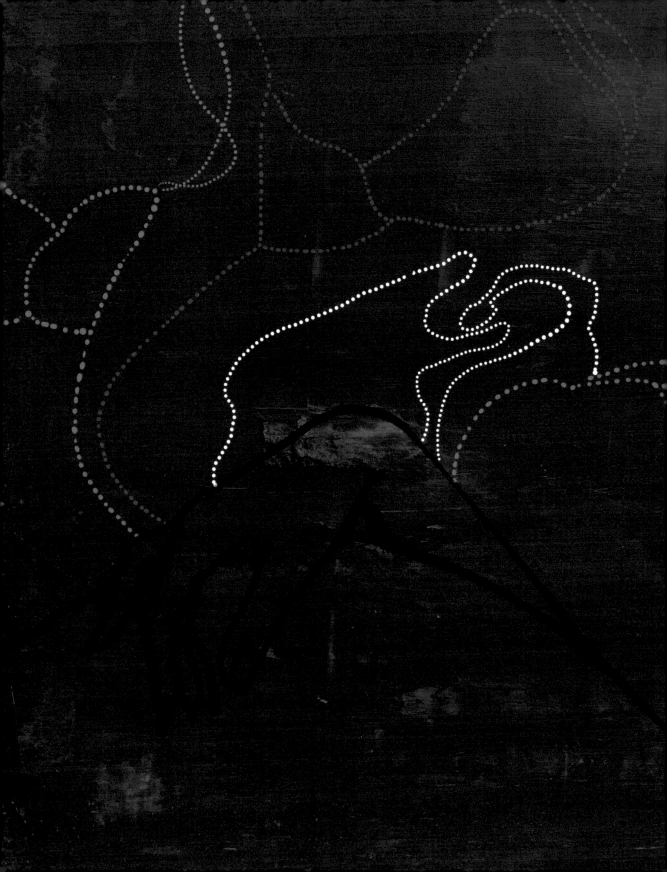

chapter three
boobs & arms

O

OVER THE CENTURIES BREASTS HAVE BEEN PUSHED UP, PULLED DOWN, FLATTENED, PARTLY EXPOSED, TOTALLY EXPOSED, HOIKED HITHER AND HAULED THITHER. NO MATTER WHAT SHAPE AND SIZE, THEY CAN BE AN ONGOING CHALLENGE FOR US WOMEN. WHAT ARE WE SUPPOSED TO DO WITH THEM? THEY'RE SUCH HYSTERICAL THINGS IF YOU THINK ABOUT THEM.

My breasts have changed shape quite a lot over the years. When I was a teenager, they were almost non-existent and my first bra (32A) I stuffed with cotton wool! It's so funny – when I didn't have boobs, I longed for them; now I do, I wouldn't mind them being smaller. But hey, they have a mind of their own, and actually lots of clothes look great with a cleavage, as long as it's not too exposed.

It's most important to wear good supporting bras, not only for looks but for comfort. For my bras I love to try lots of different labels but I do think **M&S** has some of the best and, cost-wise, is great.

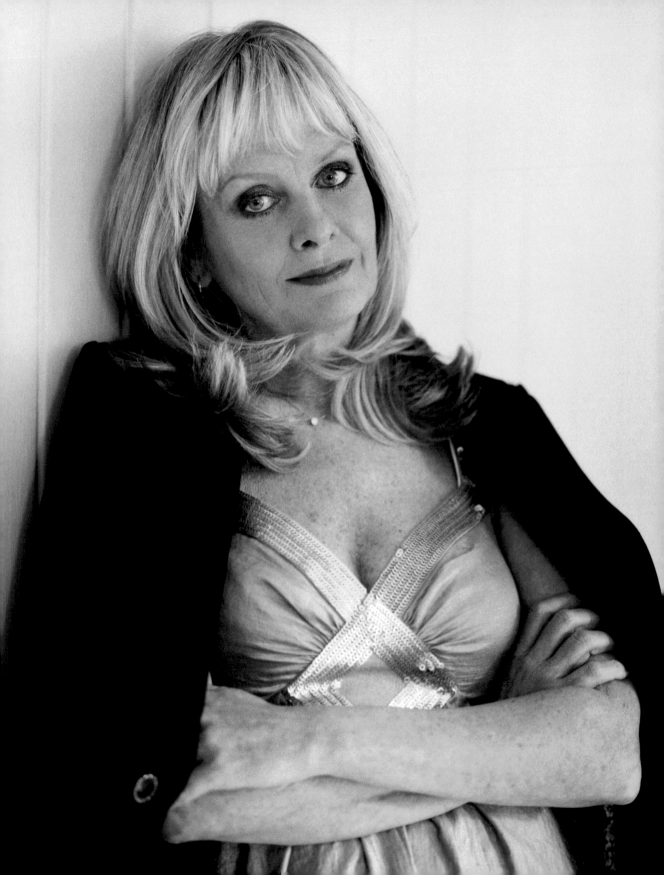

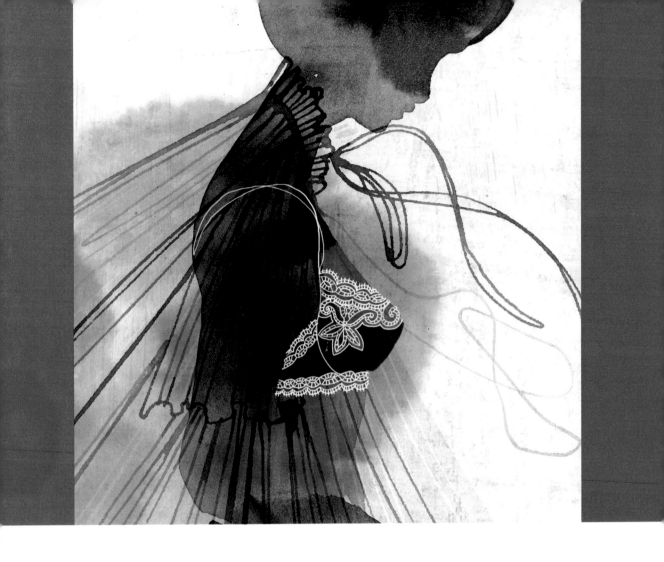

Bra fittings are always free and it is far more economical to invest in four that fit perfectly as opposed to a dozen that don't

When I look for a new bra my size can jump considerably, depending on the manufacturer. And it's not just a discrepancy on the label, it's our bodies too. That is why it is so important to have them measured every six months, or at least when you notice a change in body weight or comfort in your current underwear. Better still, always try on a bra before buying and never assume it will fit you from the label. Even if you get your boobs measured at a trusted high-street store, try each bra on first. Avoid mail order, unless you know the brand and size well.

June Kenton is the owner of **RIGBY & PELLER**, and personal corsetier to the Queen. With over two hundred drawers of underwear and stocking up to a J cup, her stores are world renowned for being the authority on proper support when it comes to our most feminine of assets.

'When you are a teenager, your breasts are full in the cup, amazingly so,' says June. 'Then, if you go on the pill, they increase in size again. When you have babies, it all goes wild and your breasts might not go back down to their original size. Not wearing the right bra for maternity causes them to drop and change shape very quickly and nothing can reverse that. Post-maternity, they drop even more as there is no muscle in the breast area. During the menopause, HRT can increase your breasts by up to one or two cup sizes. If you are not on HRT, the reverse can happen and breasts may shrink and slip down.'

The most persistent challenge to keeping our breasts perky is finding the right kind of bra to support them. Ensure you are doing this, and you can dramatically improve your body shape. Some women with bigger busts sleep in bras too. It's all about support.

'Chain stores can have their own-brand bras made by up to twelve different manufacturers, so no two bras, even same style, will be the same,' says June. If you have larger breasts, and your bra isn't giving you the correct support, then every time you walk, your skin stretches, causing stretch marks, shoulder and back problems,' she says.

According to June, the commonest mistake women make is to pull the straps tight in order to lift the breasts and make up for the lack of support. This causes shoulder and neck pain, and it can also cause a strain on the chest and even on the breathing.

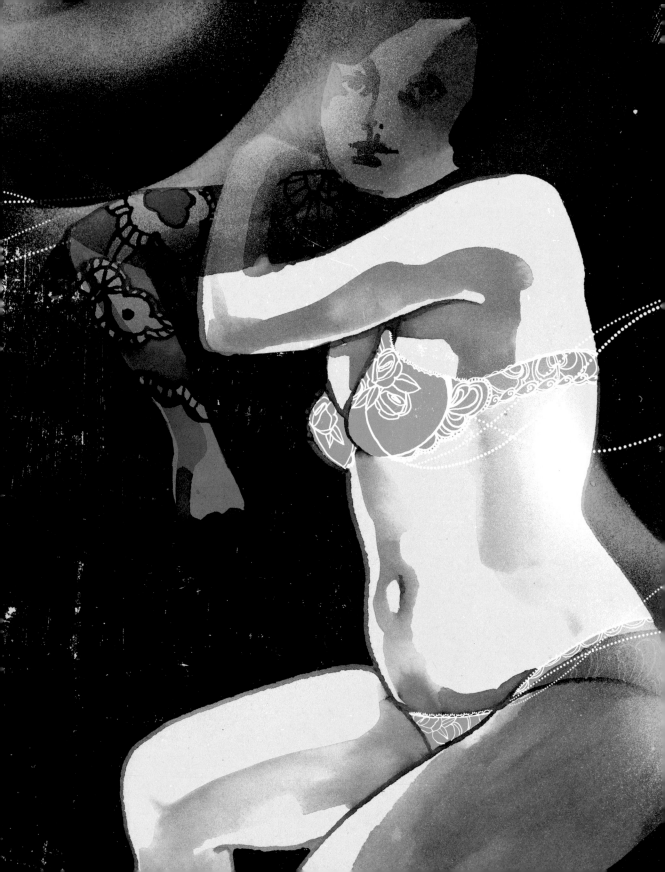

HOW TO TELL IF YOUR BRA FITS

FOR THIS SECTION I CONSULTED RIGBY & PELLER'S JUNE KENTON AND NASHEETA MASOET. ACCORDING TO THEM, A SHOCKING 85 PER CENT OF WOMEN ARE WEARING THE WRONG BRA SIZE! THANKS TO THEIR SUGGESTIONS THERE ARE NOW NO EXCUSES, GIRLS . . .

1. Stand in front of the mirror and look at how the bra is fitting you. Your breasts, no matter what their size, should not be touching. Believe it or not, they are perfectly happy on their own.

2. There should be a little gap between the breast and the underwiring. If not, then it means the bra isn't sitting on the chest wall, where it should be.

3. It should not dig in anywhere, nor should the ends be pressing into the breast itself.

4. Lift your arms up. If the bra rises up then it is the wrong size. Even when you are in the fitting room being measured by an expert, lift your arms up, touch your toes, move around a bit. The bra should work with you and not move around.

5. The back of the bra should be level with the underwiring, not riding up.

6. Most importantly, you should have two breasts, not four, and not six!

7. Put your clothes back on over the bra you are trying out. This is vital, as only then can you tell how it looks. You should have lots of bras to complement different clothes.

8. You will be amazed at how gorgeous your boobs will look in the right fitting bra.

9. When putting on your bra, put your arms through the straps and then lean forward so your breasts are falling into the bra cups, then bring them up together and fasten. This ensures your breasts are fully supported by the entirety of the bra and not just sitting in the top of it.

10. If you are wearing the correct size for the first time, it may feel tight and slightly uncomfortable to begin with. Persevere!

BRAS YOU MIGHT LIKE TO TRY

- *LEPEL – Sophisticated designs like the rose-print Pandora set. Cups are lined in a soft cotton. Available in sizes 32A to 38DD.*
- *FAYREFORM – Specifically for bigger-busted women, in lace-trimmed styles like the Opulent Underwired Plunge Bra. Available in sizes 32D to 40DD.*
- *M&S – A great selection of bras at competitive prices. What's more, you can take them home to try in sizes ranging from 30A to 44GG.*

BIG BOOBS

IF YOU HAVE LARGER BREASTS, DON'T BUY A CHEAP BRA. You simply cannot get the same quality in cheaper underwear. The elastic won't be as good, the finish won't be as smooth and the support just won't be there. Spend as much as you can afford!

PRETTY BRAS

I'VE GOT SOME M&S BRAS FROM QUITE A FEW YEARS BACK, WITH ELASTICATED VELVET STRAPS IN PRETTY HUES. In the summer it's great to wear them with dresses. If you have to show a bra strap, show a pretty one. Those ones I'll hang on to until they disintegrate. Most big department stores have a huge stock of brands. M&S is my favourite for undies and always has been. Great choice, great prices.

You really have to try a bra on. It is so bad for your body to wear the wrong size. And spend as much as you can afford!

A LITTLE BIT OF HELP FROM OUR FRIENDS

NOT ALL OF US ARE WELL ENDOWED IN THE BOSOM DEPARTMENT. THERE ARE SOME AMAZING PRODUCTS TO ENHANCE THE BUST WITHOUT RESORTING TO SURGERY.

Bust-enhancing products

FASHION FORMS – Wide selection of bras designed to be invisible under clothing. Range includes: **BANDEAU BRA, SILICONE ADHESIVE BODY BRAS, EXTREME SILICONE PLUNGE BRA** and the **NUBRA SELF-ADHESIVE SILICONE ENHANCER**.

THE NATURAL – Range of seamless nude bras and breast 'items' for outfit dilemmas. Products include **CLEARLY NATURAL** underwired strapless bra, smooth support cups, bra-strap converter, low-back converter, and the ever-popular **MAX BOOST** regular-size silicone bust enhancer.

FASHION FIRST AID – *'For when the gods of fashion decide today is not going to be your day…'* Wide range of silicone-based items that include **SUPPORTITS** adhesive bra, **BOOSTITS** full cup/half cup silicone inserts, nipple concealers, **LIFTITS** adhesive support and **TAPITS** double-sided tape.

ELIXIR – New brand of lingerie created by **LEJABY** especially for women with a fuller bust. Their underwear is feminine, and extremely comfortable and supportive. Excellent for curvaceous women. **ELIXIR** Salome Plunge Bra is a **RIGBY & PELLER** bestseller. It is supportive up to a size 36F, and is perfect for women with fuller breasts who want to look sexy. Sizes range from 30D to 38G.

BRAZA – This label developed the concept of the self-adhesive bra in 1984. Range includes **BRA ADHESIVE SUPPORTS, FASHION TAPE, MAGICUPS, PETAL TOPS** and **LOW DOWN BACK CONVERTERS**.

boobs & arms

BUST CREAMS YOU MIGHT LIKE TO TRY

LUXURY

- *Mama Mio Boob Tube*
- *Elemis Pro-Collagen Lifting Treatment for Neck and Bust*
- *Sisley Phytobuste*

MIDDLE

- *This Works Perfect Cleavage*
- *Clarins Bust Beauty Gel*
- *Bliss Thinny Thin Chin*

CALVIN KLEIN UNDERWEAR – Their bras are better for smaller-busted women. Their signature light, underwired bras and soft-cotton triangle bras are super-comfy. Sizes from 32A to 36D.

PATRICIA – Finnish lingerie and swimwear company. Due to the gentleness and flexibility of the underwire and soft delicate lace, the range is ideal for all age groups and especially post-mastectomy customers. Sizes from 30C to 38D.

PRIMA DONNA – Stocks a wide range of lingerie, appealing to women of all ages, particularly women with fuller breasts, ranging from full D cups to generous H cups. Sizes from 32D to 42H.

UNDER COVER – A naturally discreet collection of breast enhancers and bra accessories, ideal for everyday and occasional wear. Breast enhancers fit a wide range of sizes, offering suitable wear for up to a DD cup. Other UNDER COVER varieties are available in one size, suitable for all.

BUST CREAMS

YOU MIGHT ALSO LIKE TO TRY A BUST CREAM, although I'm not sure of their long-lasting effects. They do achieve temporary tightening, according to my beauty experts. They are all pricey and a real treat purchase.

bliss

thinny thin chin

for jiggly jowls and droopy décolletés

- like a liquid bra for your 'v-zone'
- tightens while targeting double-chin trouble
- improves appearance of neck lines and cleavage creases

super-strength skincare from bliss, new york's hottest spa

e 50 mL /1.7 fl oz

TOTAL FITNESS

SPRAY BUSTE ULTRA-LIFTANT
ULTRA-LIFTING BUST SPRAY

CLARINS

Elemis

PRO-COLLAGEN
LIFTING
TREATMENT

NECK AND BUST

ANTI-AGEING

50ml e 1.7 fl.oz.

arms

IF THERE'S ANYWHERE ON A WOMAN'S BODY THAT AGES IN A VERY FRUSTRATING FASHION, IT HAS TO BE THE UPPER ARMS. The skin under the upper arm can become loose. Even on the tautest, most toned creatures, armpits have been known to resemble chicken wings, and let's not even talk about bingo wings. I'm afraid these can happen with age, although arm exercises may help. So fear not. There are also plenty of tricks to help conceal what loosening and drooping there may be. One of the best tricks is ditching short-sleeved T-shirts for ones that have just-to-the-elbow sleeves, or an added cuff.

If you're going out and want to up the glam stakes without flashing the upper-arm problem areas, team a corset, bustier or strapless dress with a shrug or a sequinned shawl. I have a gorgeous black chiffon shawl which brings a certain elegance to the upper body.

You might like to try Pilates exercises for the upper arm, which I do with a couple of tins of beans or whatever's knocking about in the cupboard at home. You will need to have these taught to you by a qualified Pilates instructor. It doesn't take long and can really make a difference to reverse that floppy upper-arm feeling. To find a Pilates instructor near you, look at the following websites: **www.pilatesfoundation.com** and **www.pilates.co.uk**

Concealing the arms is sexy and becomes ever more so the older we get

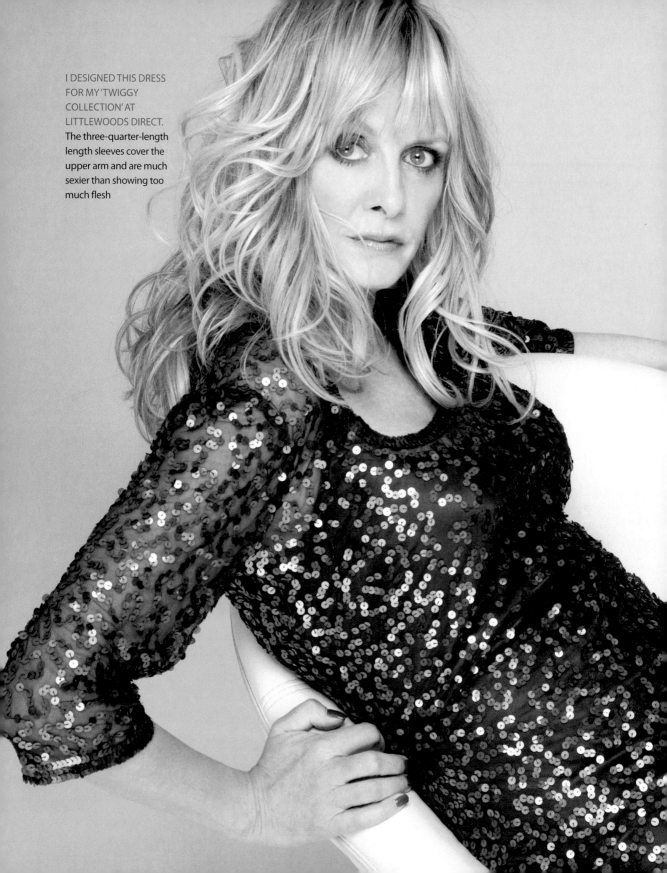

I DESIGNED THIS DRESS
FOR MY 'TWIGGY
COLLECTION' AT
LITTLEWOODS DIRECT.
The three-quarter-length
length sleeves cover the
upper arm and are much
sexier than showing too
much flesh

FIRST AID FOR ARMS

IT IS EASY TO FORGET THE BACK OF THE ARMS WHEN MOISTURIZING. Before you shower, try using a body brush on these areas too, to help circulation and thereby prevent mottled skin. Treat your arms as you would your face. Give them plenty of TLC!

Try these sleeve suggestions

1 **FLUTED SLEEVES** or any sleeve that flares out before coming in again at the wrist are very feminine and a great way to distract from the dreaded bingo wings.

2 **T-SHIRT SLEEVES THAT FALL TO JUST ABOVE OR BELOW THE ELBOW** are more flattering than the short-sleeved T-shirt shape.

3 **IF YOU WEAR A SLEEVELESS TOP,** team it with a lightweight cotton cardi left undone. You could also consider a sheer long-sleeved cotton T-shirt underneath for extra coverage.

4 **YOU CAN EVEN WEAR LONG-SLEEVED COTTON OR SILK JERSEY T-SHIRTS UNDER SLEEVELESS DRESSES.** It works really well. I have lovely strappy summer dresses, but feel uncomfortable bearing my under-arm area. Light layering underneath is a modern alternative to a cardi for coverage.

5 **JUICY COUTURE MATERNITY T-SHIRTS.** Maternity T-shirts can be fantastic as they are longer and cut higher under the arms than regular ones, enabling you to wear a structured bra without flashing it to the world.

T-SHIRTS

T-SHIRTS ARE SO MUCH A PART OF OUR WARDROBES, BUT AS WE GET OLDER SOME OF THE SHAPES ARE LESS EASY TO WEAR. Beware boxy-shaped T-shirts as these can accentuate any upper-arm issues you may have. I know this might sound obvious but if you don't like your arms, cover them up. Stretchy T-shirts with tons of Lycra work very well as a base layer, but beware of too much stretch. Personally, I prefer one 100 per cent cotton Ts. They are kinder to lumps and bumps than figure-hugging ones and feel nicer against the skin.

If you are buying high-street T-shirts, it's often worth going a size bigger as they tend to shrink in the wash. Why are so many T-shirts so stingy on the length? Call me old fashioned, but I'd rather wear my pyjamas outside the house than be flashing my kidney area due to a short, riding-up top.

Extra-long-sleeved T-shirts are a lifesaver for me. I wear them so often, either underneath a shirt with the sleeve pulled out of the cuff, or underneath gypsy tops, tunic tops and waistcoats. I love to layer a very fine-cotton, long-sleeved T-shirt underneath a tunic top, dress or something quite loose fitting. Worn in this way, I feel comfortable dressing in tops which might otherwise feel a bit too young. The trick is to hunt out fine cotton. Anything too thick and dense can add on a pound or two to the overall silhouette.

The most flattering shape for T-shirts can be a V-neck. If it is too plunging on the cleavage, you could always layer it underneath with a simple white vest or camisole.

The length of T-shirts can be the difference between a great outfit and real disaster

boobs & arms

151

TOP T-SHIRT SHOPPING TIPS

- **VERTICAL RIBBING ON T-SHIRTS IS A GOOD CHOICE.** It can be slimming and doesn't ruck up like other cotton.
- **THICKER COTTON GIVES THE BEST COVERAGE,** whereas sheer-cotton Ts are a window straight through to bra details and bulges. Sheer is very unforgiving even on the most perfect figure, so avoid it unless you are using it as a base layer.
- **EVEN IF YOUR BOSOMS ARE YOUR BEST ASSET,** deep round-neck or scoop-neck T-shirts can be too revealing. Offset this flash of gorgeousness by covering up your arms with a little cardi that has sleeves to the elbow.
- **UNLESS YOU ARE RATHER FLAT CHESTED** and don't need to wear bras, shallow scoop-neck Ts can give you a mono-boob.
- **BUTTON-FRONT GRANDAD TS ARE GREAT.** Often a better fit, they tend to use more fabric in the places you need, such as around your middle, and are therefore more versatile. Button them up to be prim, layer them with a shirt/cardi/jacket, or button them down for an alternative to evening layers.
- **V-NECKS ARE GREAT FOR ALL BODY SHAPES AND SIZES.**

You can buy great <u>*T-shirts*</u> *at*

- <u>AMERICAN APPAREL</u> – plain T-shirts with good sleeve and body length, but be careful of sizing as they cut them very small.

- <u>C AND C CALIFORNIA</u> – good lengths, and they keep their shape over time.

- <u>GAP</u> – easy colours in fine cotton.

- <u>UNIQLO</u> – super value and great colours, perfect with slim jeans for weekend wear.

- <u>M&S</u> – great for layering, they wash and wear really well and are also excellent value.

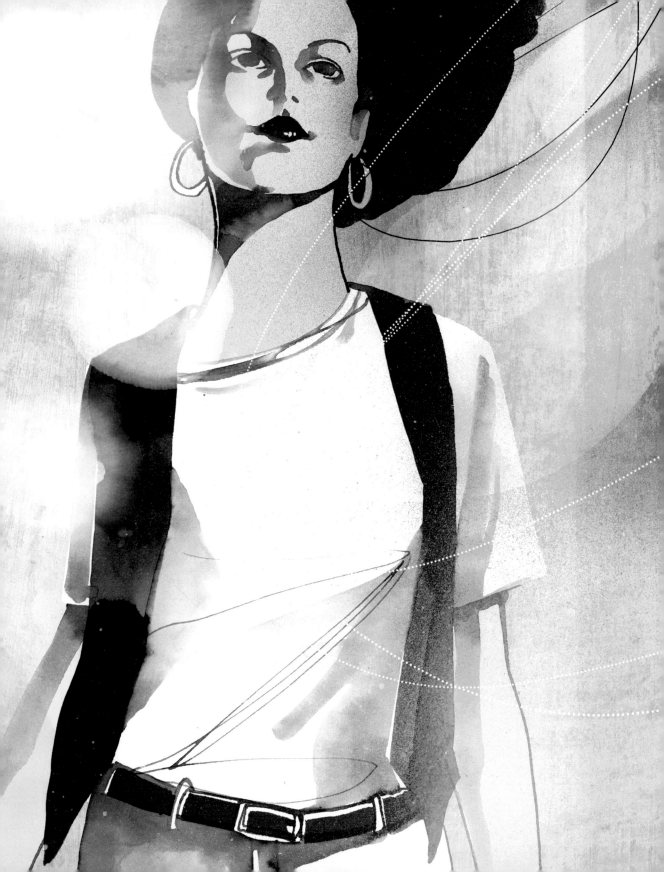

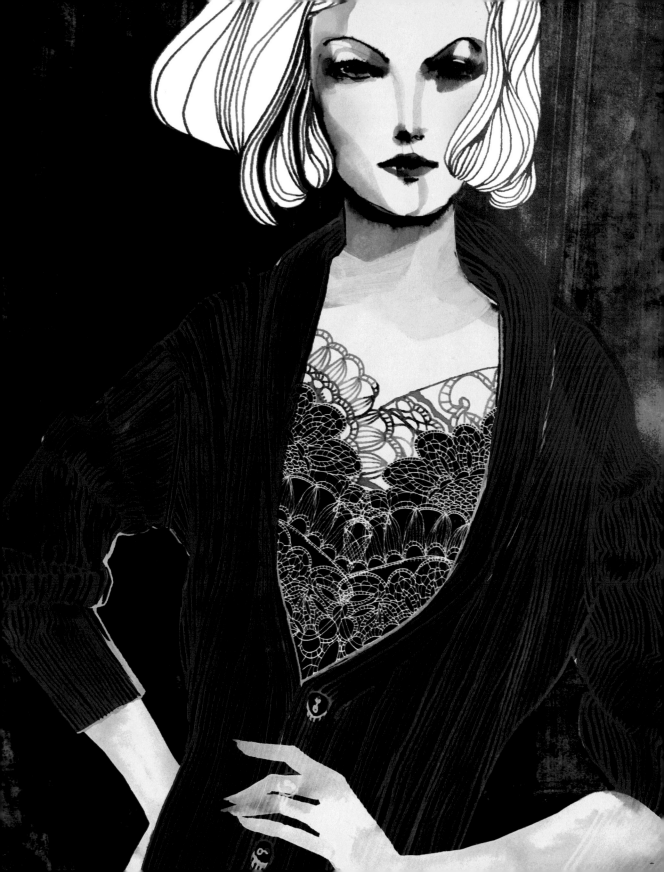

KNITWEAR

WHETHER YOU ARE A CARDIGAN GIRL OR A SWEATER FIEND, KNITWEAR IS ESSENTIAL AND CAN PLAY A VITAL PART IN LAYERING. In the olden days, us girls would have worn twinset cardigans with a matching short-sleeved top in the same fabric underneath. Nowadays, the simplicity of a lightweight cardigan makes it one of the best ways to layer outfits. Even in the summer, a light cotton cardi can be a girl's best friend. It is ideal for concealing the upper arms and can be worn either snugly, with one button done up at the top, or simply left open, even if you're wearing a belt cinched at the waist. I love grandad cardis for winter, worn over a vintage lace shirt, waistcoat and full skirt with slouchy boots.

NOA NOA is another of the Danish wonder labels (like **DAY BIRGER ET MIKKELSEN**) that offers women casualwear at competitive prices. For summer, their crisp cotton dresses and shirts are wardrobe staples, whilst for winter, the chunky knits and wide leg trousers are wonderfully snug and super-comfortable.

The Cardigan Glossary

• *TWINSET CARDIS*
Good for concealing upper-arm problem areas.

• *V-NECK, THREE-BUTTON GRANDAD CARDIS*
Good for layering over jeans if your tummy protrudes, but be sure to button them unless you are wearing a shirt untucked or something else is covering the waistband. Also lovely thrown on over casual clothes at weekends.

• *LONG CARDIS WITH BELT*
Good for concealing big tums, wide hips and bums, especially on taller shapes. Avoid wearing with wide trousers; they work much better with full skirts or jeans.

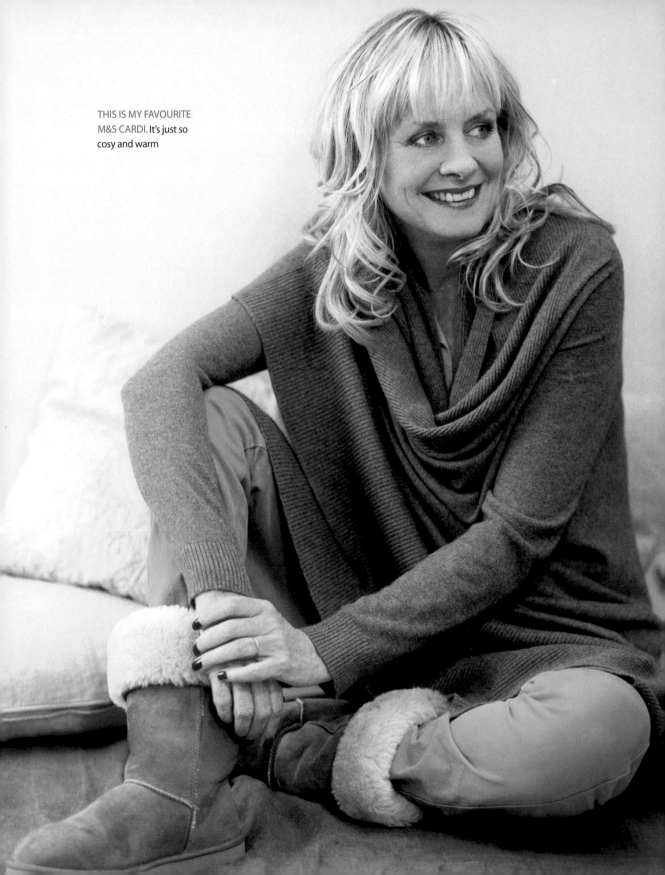

THIS IS MY FAVOURITE
M&S CARDI. It's just so
cosy and warm

You can buy great <u>knitwear</u> at

- <u>**TOAST**</u> – Great chunky knits for throwing on over outfits; always really nice shapes and styles. They also do great tops and thinner knitwear for layering.

- <u>**PURE COLLECTION**</u> – Online and mail-order cashmere company, specializing in a wide range of basics. Best collections are the **MODERN CLASSICS** and **SOFTLY SOFTLY**, with something to suit all shapes and sizes. They also do a women's **SUPERFINE CASHMERE** range which is great under jackets.

- <u>**FLORENCE & FRED (TESCO)**</u> – Good classic shapes, with a wide selection of colours. Generous in length. They also do a very nice, fine, cable-knit cashmere sweater.

- <u>**M&S**</u> – Their cashmere is fabulous and they do great winter woollies, cardis and summery cotton knits too.

- <u>**UNIQLO**</u> – This Japanese high-street label stocks cheap, good-quality fleeces, cardigans and cashmere sweaters in amazing colour ranges.

- <u>**JIGSAW**</u> – Consistently stocks an extensive range of wrap/tie/cropped cardigans, often with pretty detailing on the buttons and in lots of colours. The seasonal colours, like the purples, greens and burgundy in the winter, are a great investment to update your wardrobe.

boobs & arms

- **AGNÈS B** – Classic and petite in design, these cardigans come in a range of basic, practical colours perfect for layering with a simple shirt for work. Not suitable for women with a larger bust due to the narrow fit, but lovely for all ages. Great range of different styles each season.

- **COMPTOIR DES COTONNIERS** – This French high-street label's cardigans and wraps are cut with lots of fabric. Garments have an ageless appeal. The fabric hangs well and is flattering on the tummy.

- **JOSEPH** – The price points from this store are a little higher than high-street prices, but the store's own label can be very trend led, and is always well cut. Long-length black cardigans in cashmere and merino wool are a staple from season to season. Long, buttonless wraps suitable for a larger figure and bust are a great investment, well worth splurging on!

- **DKNY** – This diffusion line specializes in knitwear and wraps. Another good range for layering is DKNY PURE: a collection of fine white and neutral cottons designed for casual daywear and slouching around at home. Every item can pretty much be layered with another. Excellent for all shapes and sizes.

- **KEW** – Sister company of JIGSAW, with similar styles of cardis but lower price points. Best buys are long open cardigans with tie waists, a wide-rib tonal lace cardigan and the shorter cotton-cashmere tie cardigan. All come in a selection of seasonal colours.

- **WHISTLES** – Every season this high-street chain does a button-front knit dress that works really well over jeans, giving a very slimming silhouette. Their cardigans have plenty of fabric with a deep scoop neckline and fluted shapes that skim just below the knee. Cotton wraps are a good alternative to the higher-priced equivalents. If you have a big bust stay away from their sweater dresses, and from their signature bright jazzy prints.

- **MONSOON** – Their sleeveless cable cardigan is a brilliant item for layering, as well as having a tie waist to emphasize shape. Monsoon also stocks a brilliant selection of shrugs each season that work well with party dresses and sleeveless tops.

hands

A LOT OF WOMEN REALLY TAKE CARE OF THEMSELVES AND THEIR FACES, FORGETTING TO GIVE THEIR HANDS THE SAME AMOUNT OF ATTENTION. If you haven't worn washing-up gloves since you were a teenager, chances are your hands will be significantly more lined and mottled than the rest of your body. The way around this is to moisturize as much as possible, and keep hand creams beside your bed, in your handbag and at the kitchen and bathroom sink. During the day, wear a hand cream with sun-protection in it as your hands are almost always exposed to skin-damaging UV light.

For a treat, there's nothing quite as soothing as a warm paraffin-wax hand treatment. It is intensely moisturizing and helps reduce swelling in joints, soothes pain from arthritis and tendonitis, and improves circulation.

As we get older, circulation can become weaker. If you keep blood circulating properly to your hands, they will keep getting the nutrients. Facialist and beauty guru **EVE LOM** suggests piano lessons are a wonderful way to exercise the hands.

Look out for creams that contain mulberry root, known to help tackle liver spots, as well as kojic and ascorbic acid. 'My grandmother used to use lemon juice, which helped lighten her hands a bit,' says Dr David Colbert. 'Just don't use it in the summer as it can react with the sun.' Also, if you are having a peel or laser on your face, ask them to do your hands as well. It is important to keep an eye on moles and liver spots on the hands that may develop as you get older.

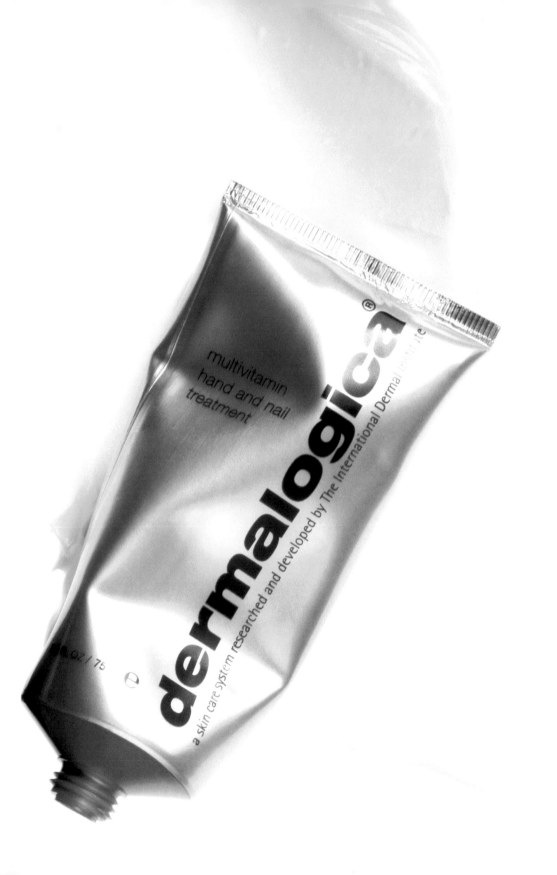

If you notice anything that seems raised, or is itchy/uncomfortable/irregular, visit your GP or, better still, visit a dermatologist. It might just be a liver spot. This can be treated either with cryotherapy, which freezes off the spot by creating a blister that peels off after one week, or with a 35 per cent TCA spot treatment peel. Make sure you cover the area afterwards as it'll be more sensitive to sunlight.

NAILS

I USED TO BITE MY NAILS UNTIL I WAS ABOUT TWENTY AND, AS A RESULT, THEY ARE VERY THIN AND WEAK AND BREAK EASILY. About ten years ago, I did a shampoo commercial which required a close-up shot of my hands. The manicurist on the shoot recommended I have them wrapped with silk fibre, and I have been doing this ever since. A thin piece of fabric is applied to the nail and a liquid resin is then added on top. I do this every two weeks I prefer short nails to long talons. **ELEGANCE BEAUTY CLINIC** in London is excellent for nail wraps, manicures and pedicures. They also do an extensive range of beauty treatments such as radio frequency and laser.

If you're going for an evening out, try to get your nails painted. If you go to all the trouble of wearing a posh frock, tatty old nails look horrible. It's beautiful to see an older woman with gorgeous hands, nails and jewels. But you don't have to travel to London for great nails. Check your local beauty salon, and be sure to get a personal recommendation.

HAND CREAMS YOU MIGHT LIKE TO TRY

LUXURY

- *Elemis Pro-collagen Hand and Nail Cream*
- *Dior Capture Totale Multi-Perfection Hand Repair Creme SPF 15*
- *Eve Lom Hand Cream with SPF 10*

MIDDLE

- *Dermalogica Multivitamin Hand and Nail Treatment*
- *Jurlique Lavender Hand Cream*

BUDGET

- *L'Occitane Cherry Blossom Petal-Soft Hand Cream*

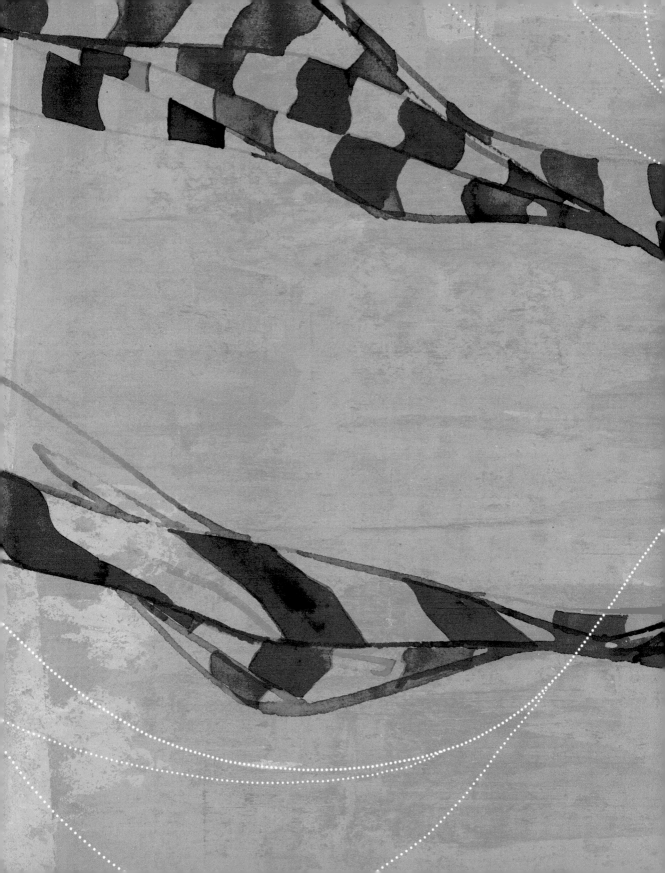

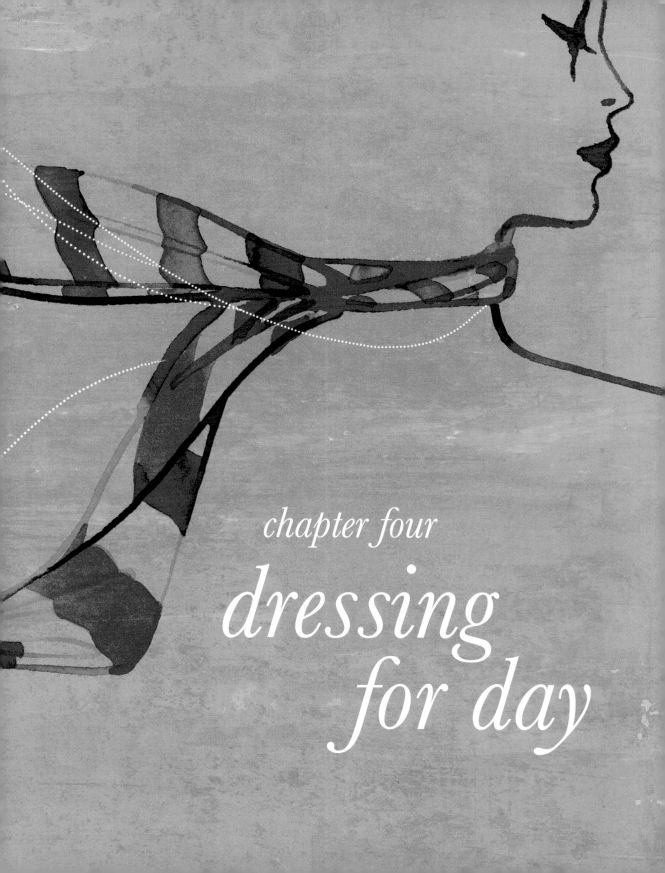

chapter four

dressing for day

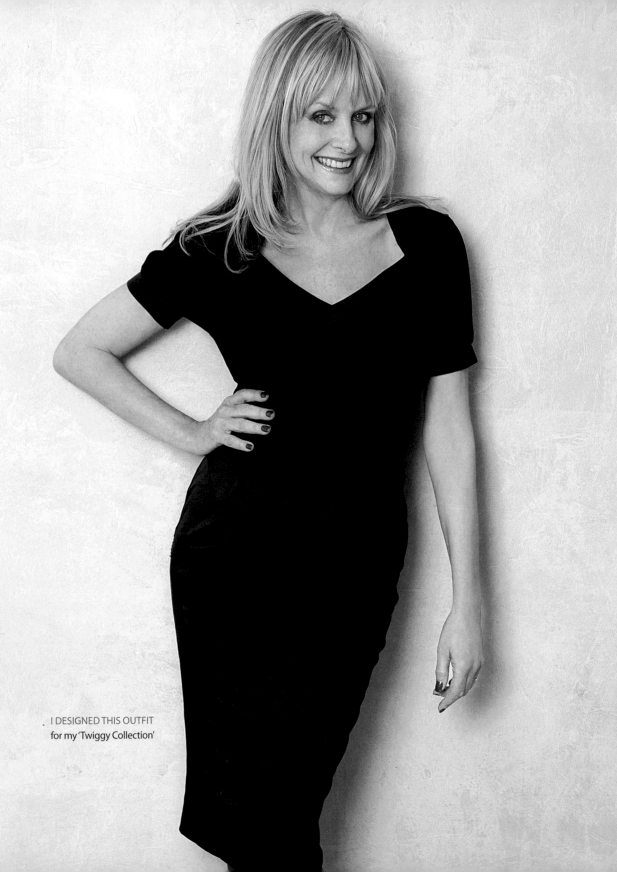

I DESIGNED THIS OUTFIT
for my 'Twiggy Collection'

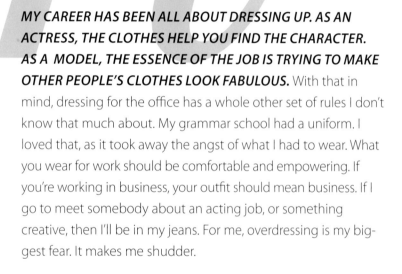

MY CAREER HAS BEEN ALL ABOUT DRESSING UP. AS AN ACTRESS, THE CLOTHES HELP YOU FIND THE CHARACTER. AS A MODEL, THE ESSENCE OF THE JOB IS TRYING TO MAKE OTHER PEOPLE'S CLOTHES LOOK FABULOUS. With that in mind, dressing for the office has a whole other set of rules I don't know that much about. My grammar school had a uniform. I loved that, as it took away the angst of what I had to wear. What you wear for work should be comfortable and empowering. If you're working in business, your outfit should mean business. If I go to meet somebody about an acting job, or something creative, then I'll be in my jeans. For me, overdressing is my biggest fear. It makes me shudder.

One of my close girlfriends runs a business in the City. She invests in key accessories to elevate her everyday uniform of a sharply tailored power suit. If she's going straight from the office to an evening do, she adds a piece of costume jewellery such as a sparkly brooch to her lapel, upgrades her shirt to a sequinned tunic top – and *voilà*! I love seeing a woman work a strict dominatrix suit, complete with pencil skirt, heels and a man's shirt.

dressing for day

TIPS FOR OFFICE CHIC

I CONSULTED A HANDFUL OF EXPERTS WHO KNOW MORE THAN A THING OR TWO ABOUT DRESSING FOR WORK: DESIGNERS SIR PAUL SMITH AND BETTY JACKSON, BOUTIQUE OWNER MRS B, FROM BROWNS, AND CITY BOUTIQUE OWNER MADELEINE HAMILTON.

- **DRESS FOR YOUR AGE**. Don't try hard to be younger if it is inappropriate. Know your character and personality, and dress accordingly.

- **BE PRACTICAL.** If you travel a lot, comfortable clothes are really important. Go for clothes you can move in, clothes that have pockets and clothes that don't need laundering or pressing every few minutes.

- *DRESSING FOR WORK DEPENDS ON WHAT YOUR WORK IS. If you are a lawyer, say, or you work in accountancy or are head of a business, keep it simple. Good quality but not too sexy will always pay dividends in the workplace.*

- **RESEARCH THE SHOP OR SHOPS BEFORE YOU GO.** Follow recommendations of colleagues. Seek out independents where a more personal service is the norm, if your budget allows.

- **SELECT PRACTICAL FABRICS,** i.e. not linen that creases immediately. Instead, go for good-quality lightweight wools.

dressing for day

166

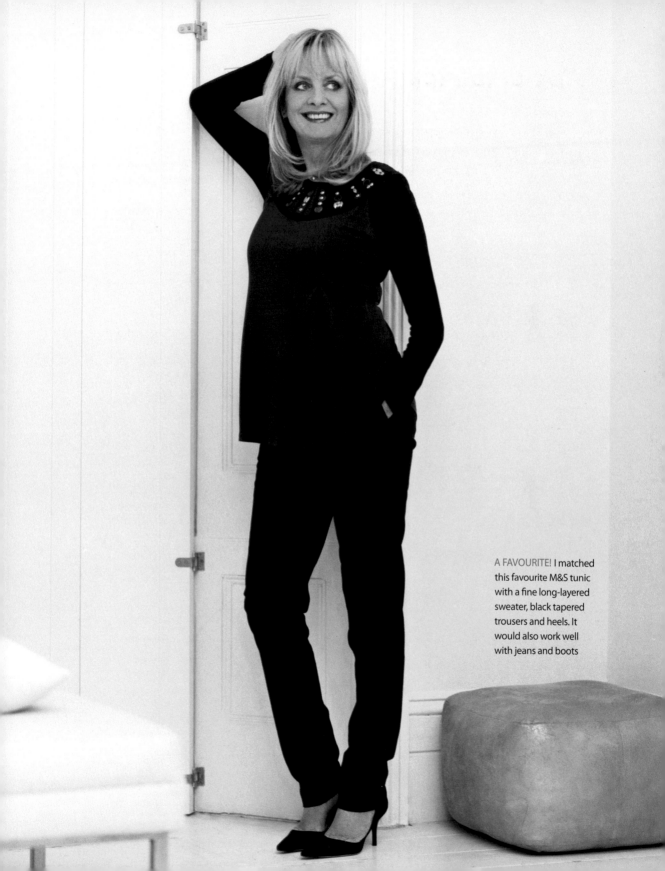

A FAVOURITE! I matched this favourite M&S tunic with a fine long-layered sweater, black tapered trousers and heels. It would also work well with jeans and boots

Invest in at least one dark-coloured, well-tailored, two-piece suit for summer and the same for winter

- **A TAILORED GARMENT CAN HELP YOU LOOK SLIMMER, TALLER AND MORE ELEGANT.** A low single-button jacket can give a longer appearance worn by shorter women.

- *CHOOSE YOUR JACKET LENGTH CAREFULLY. If you have bigger hips, hunt down a jacket that covers them.*

- **WHEN PICKING OUT TROUSERS,** a slim-legged trouser is generally more flattering than a wide leg unless you have exceptionally long limbs.

- *THINK ABOUT WHAT YOU ARE DOING AFTER WORK; remember to pop a sparkly top or a higher-heel shoe in your work bag.*

- **CHECK OUT WHETHER ALTERATIONS ARE FREE** and how long they take. Very few women walk into a ready-to-wear collection of any price level at all without some little tweaks here and there.

Leave time aside in your dressing routine for hair and make-up. It's almost as important as the suit

● **WHEN PLANNING AND PURCHASING A WORK OUTFIT**, it is important to feel comfortable and at ease with your shopping environment. There is nothing more stressful than worrying about a meeting you might be late for, or a car on a timed meter. Put time aside for your own shopping.

● **STYLES DO NOT HAVE TO BE COMPLETELY FASHION LED**, but don't shun contemporary looks. Be guided by helpful sales staff as to whether it works for you. Yes, such people exist, otherwise small boutiques would not get such repeat custom.

● *ALWAYS CHOOSE A NATURAL FIBRE such as wool for suiting. Time after time it lasts longer, looks better and, if it has some elastane or Lycra content (no more than 5 per cent), fits even better!*

● **THINK FEET FIRST. IF YOU HAVE TO SPEND A LONG TIME ON YOUR FEET, PLAN SHOES.** You may find this dictates the outfit, as comfy flats don't always work with a skirt!

dressing for day

169

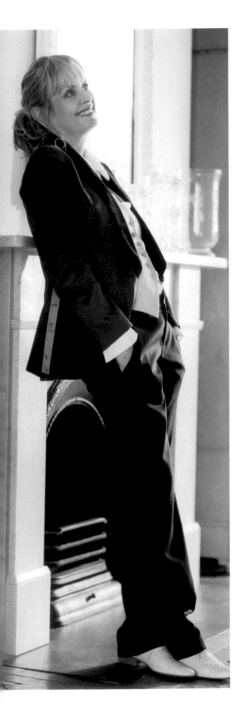

Great <u>office</u> gear to try . . .

1. Suits & separates

- **<u>BETTY JACKSON</u>** – one of the UK's most wearable designers

- **<u>BROWNS</u>** – one of the best all-round boutiques for investment pieces

- **<u>EVANS</u>** – excellent-value work wear for plus sizes, including suits and separates

- **<u>HOBBS</u>** – classic work shirts, skirts and dress suiting; skirt lengths are mostly cut below the knee and their wide-leg trousers are ultra-flattering and functional

- **<u>JAEGER</u>** – modern classic suiting for executive women, with stylish dress shirts and pinstripes

- **<u>KAREN MILLEN</u>** – good for sexy office wear, with plenty of choice when it comes to pencil skirts, fitted shirts and jackets

- **<u>L. K. BENNETT</u>** – stylish trouser and skirt suits, often in vibrant colours like green, red and blue, in addition to classic linen tweeds

- **<u>M&S</u>** – great basics: fitted shirts, A-line and pencil skirts, trouser suits, all in classic colours that wash and wear well

- **<u>MADELEINE HAMILTON</u>** – chic City store in London targeting business women, with a fantastic website

- **<u>NEXT</u>** – build up a fantastic work wardrobe with their separates and oversized jackets

- **<u>MARGARET HOWELL</u>** – excellent for trouser suits in soft cotton, corduroy or linen

- **<u>NICOLE FARHI</u>** – modern classic suiting for executive women, with stylish dress shirts and pinstripes

- **<u>PAUL SMITH</u>** – classic, sleek and sharp, the Paul Smith Black label specializes in simple but well-cut suiting, fitted blazers and tailored trousers in fine-wool flannel and chalk stripes

- **<u>PRINCIPLES</u>** – well-cut and reasonably priced trouser suits, formal suit jackets, blouses and pencil skirts

- **<u>SAVILE ROW COMPANY</u>** – excellent for formal skirt and trouser suits, and knitwear. Available online

- **<u>T. M. LEWIN</u>** – great-quality and excellent-value shirts and formal business suits, perfect for City workers

- **<u>VIYELLA</u>** – excellent-quality traditional trouser suits, bias-cut wool skirts, fitted cotton shirts, blouses and knitwear; extremely flattering and comfortable

2. Shirts

- **<u>THOMAS PINK</u>** – the classic shirtmakers – their City shirts and slim-fit shirts are excellent; they also offer a great range of cufflinks, shirt dresses and high-quality knitwear, perfect for office use

- **<u>CHARLES TYRWHITT</u>** – traditional Jermyn Street shirtmakers – their striped cotton-twill shirts for women are superb

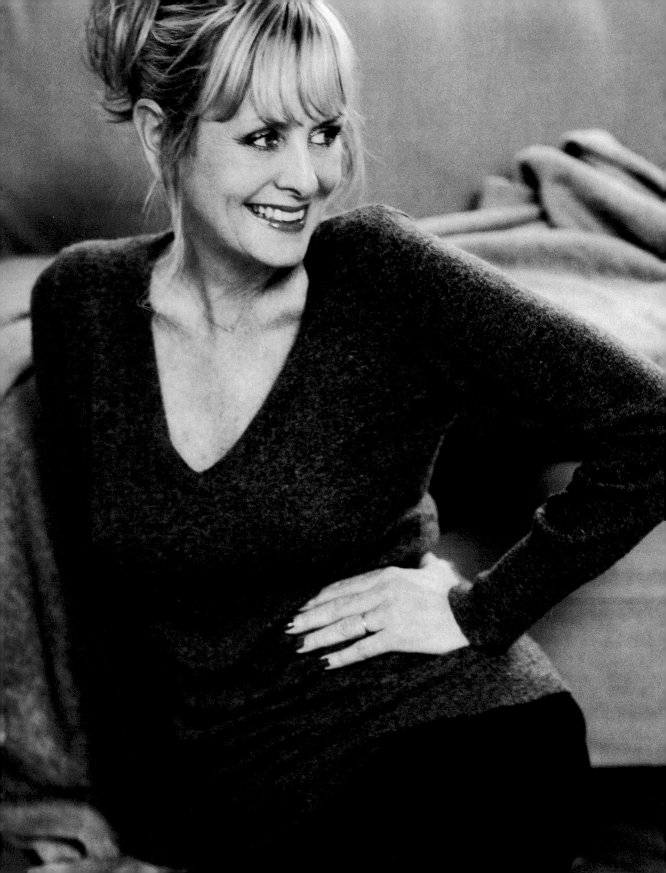

DAYTIME DRESSING

FOR THOSE OF US WHO DON'T WORK IN OFFICES, DAYTIME DRESSING HAS ITS OWN SET OF RULES. For me, it's about comfort and wearing clothes that make me feel good. You'll see evidence of my approach to daytime dressing in the pictures in this chapter. I love the mannish look – trousers, waistcoat and tailored jacket with flat, lace-up shoes. Still, that morning conundrum of having a wardrobe full of clothes but not a clue what to wear is something we all suffer from!

Great stores for <u>daywear</u> essentials

- **<u>A.P.C.</u>** – modern but classic French mail-order company specializing in great-quality cotton separates, macs, knitwear and tailored trousers

- **<u>BODEN</u>** – for easy weekend dressing, this mail-order company is so user friendly and their garments wash and wear brilliantly, with plenty of bright colours on offer

- **<u>COMPTOIR DES COTONNIERS</u>** – classic French label, perfect for loosely tailored separates and pretty but unobtrusive cotton dresses, jackets and trousers

- **<u>JIGSAW</u>** – for stylish cotton linen jackets, loose trousers and fine-knit cardigans

- **<u>JOSEPH</u>** – a little pricey but definitely worth investing in their slouchy oversize sweaters and chunky knits

- **<u>LITTLEWOODS DIRECT</u>** – check out my 'Twiggy Collection' line of clothes

- **<u>M&S</u>** – look out for smart purchases from the Autograph and Limited Collection ranges: great knitwear, women's wool trousers and shirts at fantastic prices

- **<u>TOAST</u>** – the classic easy-weekend-wear label; luxuriously simple drawstring trousers, oversize linen shirts, cotton knits and cashmere socks

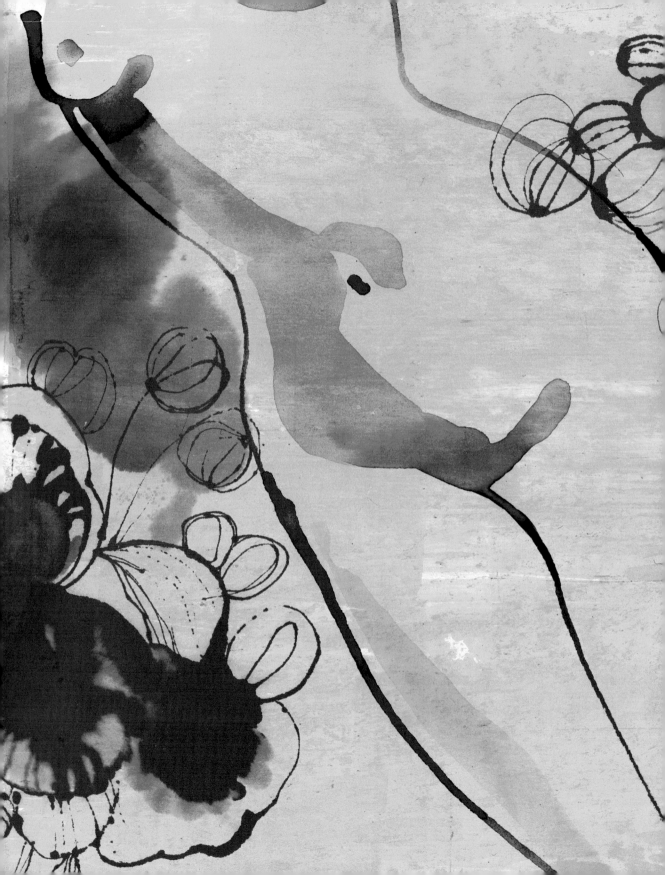

in the middle

b

BY THE TIME YOU'VE LIVED ON THE PLANET FOR HALF A CENTURY, YOU'LL HAVE COME TO ACCEPT CERTAIN THINGS ABOUT YOUR BODY. THE SHAPE OF YOUR HIPS, YOUR BONE STRUCTURE; WHETHER YOU'RE PETITE, TALL, STATUESQUE OR SMALL, THESE THINGS ARE UNCHANGEABLE.

How your body has evolved depends in my opinion more on genetics than lifestyle. It's the one you were born with. Love it for being unique to you. Chances are, there is at least one thing about your appearance you do love. Yet, all too often, women are overly critical of themselves. Ask a woman what she would like to change about her body, and she'll list a thousand things. Ask that same woman's lover/boyfriend/husband/partner and chances are he'll say he adores everything about her. Cellulite, broken veins and other physical imperfections can knock the confidence of the most beautiful women.

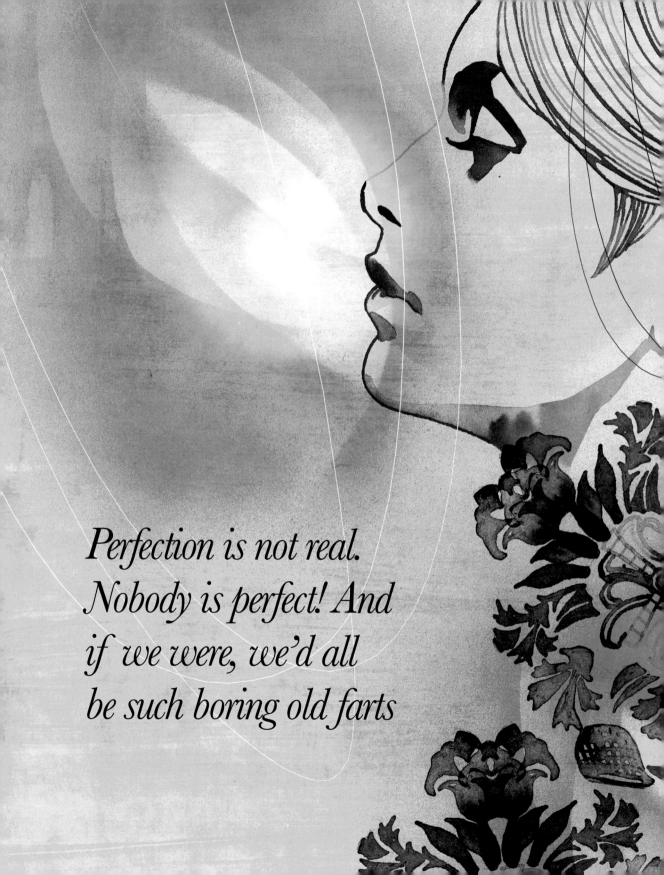

*Perfection is not real.
Nobody is perfect! And
if we were, we'd all
be such boring old farts*

There's no point in subscribing to the way a super-curvy woman dresses if your body shape is the polar opposite

Vanity and pressure to look perfect can become an unhealthy obsession in this lookist world. Next time you examine your face and body up close, inspecting every pore, every lump and every bump, remember that the only person who is scrutinizing those bits you loathe so heavily is yourself. So take a step back from that mirror, girls. Smile at your reflection. Focus on the good bits. On the inside and out, you are beautiful.

Whatever shape you are, what *is* important is to find your natural weight and size and celebrate it by dressing in a way that enhances the gorgeous bits and conceals the not-so-good lumps, bumps and bulges. Who wants to dress the same as everybody else anyway?

Most women's bodies change as time passes and I have learned to adapt the way I dress around these changes. I know I can't wear certain things any more. But you know what? That's OK. Accept it and work out what does suit your body. Chances are, there's plenty of choice out there.

If you are conscious of your tummy but you want to wear a figure-hugging skirt, rather than panic, go for black or navy, with tummy-flattening knickers. Dark colours are nearly always more flattering. Start veering into pale pinks, whites and beiges and you're instantly going to run the risk of doubling in size. Instead of feeling stressed out by having a bigger tummy zone than you'd wish for, getting stuck in a rut and dressing for comfort at the expense of looking fab – though I'm all for comfort – there are still ways of dressing without resorting to elasticated frumpwear.

Tummy-flattening knickers to buy

- **SPANX** These create a smooth line under your clothing and give you the shape you want, eliminating VPL . Expect them to feel tight!

- **MIRACLESUIT** This American-based company's claim to fame is their promise that women will look ten pounds lighter in ten seconds when wearing their products. This they achieve by using a fabric called **MIRATEX®**. They stock a wide range of control lingerie and swimwear.

- **MAIDENFORM** Fab control underwear, which is nearly always slimming and gives a flattering fit.

- **M&S** Their own-label control knickers are great! I have tons of pairs. Try the MAGIC FIRM CONTROL RIBBED KNICKERS. Their high waisted knickers with legs are a must under tight skirts.

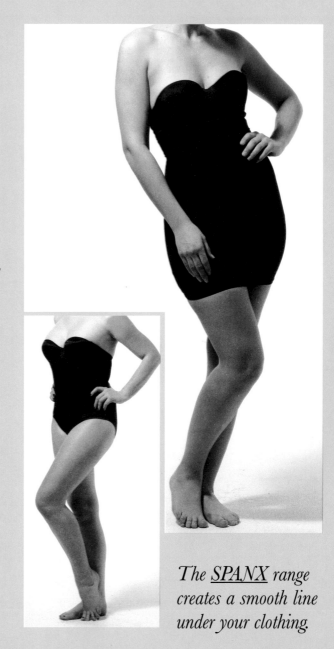

The SPANX range creates a smooth line under your clothing.

A WORD ABOUT LAYERING

LAYERING IS SO IMPORTANT. I MENTION IT IN OTHER CHAPTERS IN THIS BOOK. I've done it for years. It enables you to hide the bits you don't like, or want to draw the eye away from. For instance, I love to wear waistcoats. If you wear them with tight jeans and a T-shirt tucked in, it emphasizes your tummy too much. Instead, wear a waistcoat with the jeans and layer it with a lovely shirt to below the crotch, untucked. Let's be honest, there are very few women at any age who can wear tight, completely tucked-in things.

Rather than feeling the pressure to dress tightly, embrace softer lines, wear something velvety and luscious or add another layer to your look. It's one of the ways in which you can create a clever optical illusion.

OPTICAL ILLUSIONS

I'VE NEVER REALLY HAD A WAIST. EVEN WHEN I WAS AT MY SLIMMEST, MY SILHOUETTE WAS VERY STRAIGHT UP, STRAIGHT DOWN. But I have learned how to give myself a bit of waist by optical illusion. For this, bring on the belts.

Worn well, belts distract the eye away from a bloated tummy, a heavy-set upper body and all manner of sins. I have tons of belts, some old favourites, others recent high-street finds. They can be a superb way to update your wardrobe without breaking the bank and there's no reason to stop wearing them, EVER!

in the middle

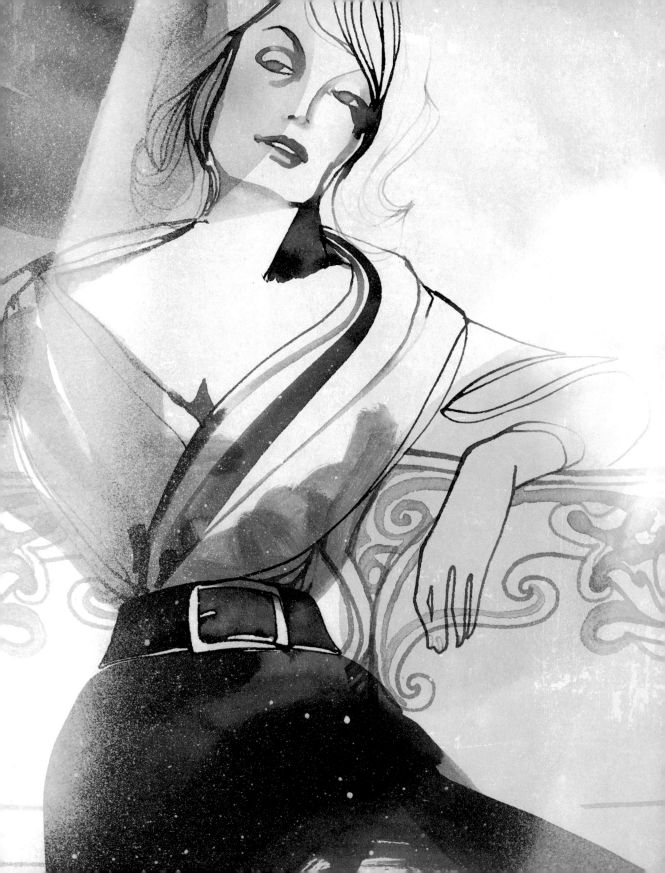

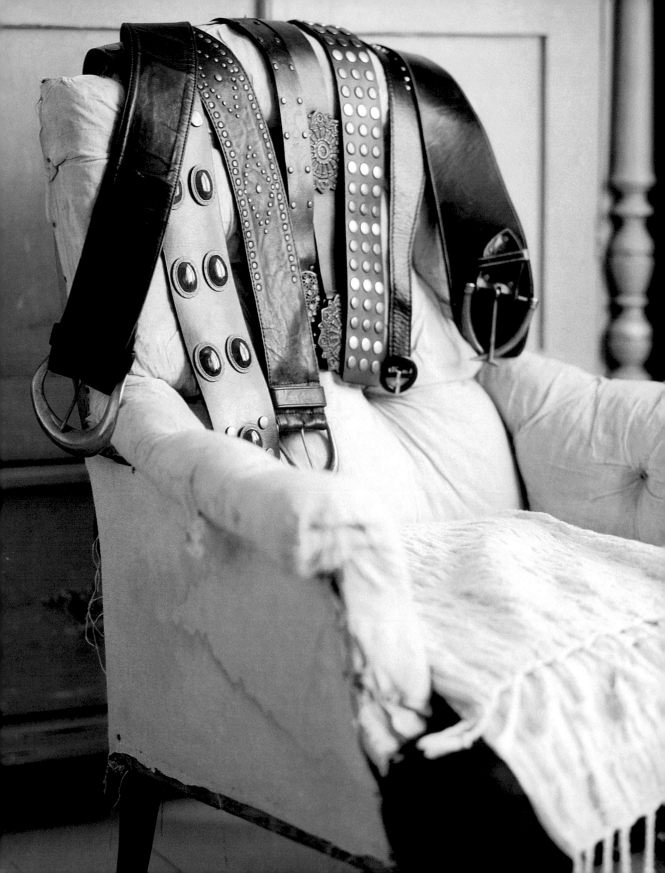

Belt up!

1 **BELTS WITH A BIT OF DECORATION/ORNAMENT ARE VERY SLIMMING.** Thin belts are great with tailored trousers.

2 **WEAR A SKIRT AND TOP WITH NO BELT** and your eyes go to the whole silhouette.

3 **A BELT VISUALLY CUTS THE OVERALL SHAPE IN HALF AND MAGICALLY MAKES FOR A MORE SLIMMING OPTICAL ILLUSION.** You don't have to be a skinny bean. Belts can be one of the kindest accessories. What's more, they don't have to cost a fortune. I have one covered in studs all the way round, with poppers that let me cinch it in for a tight fit around my waist, or loosen to wear on the hips. It is fab and cost me less than a tenner.

4 **CHUNKY BELTS CINCHED AT THE WAIST** enhance womanly curves, even on fuller figures.

5 **WITH JEANS, HIPSTER BELTS ARE GREAT WORN ON TOP OF A BIG SHIRT OR SWEATER,** but beware of overspill. If you have floppy tummy muscles this look is best avoided. However, the same kind of belt works wonders on big, billowy dresses. Rather than wearing it tightly, pull a few inches of the dress length up and inside the belt to create a flattering, tummy-concealing look.

6 **NEXT TIME YOU WEAR A SHIRT WITH TROUSERS,** consider leaving the shirt untucked, teamed with a hipster belt. This can also work with a belt cinched at the waist. Make sure the shirt is crisp.

JACKETS

WHATEVER YOUR BODY SHAPE, A TAILORED JACKET IS ONE OF THE CLEVEREST GARMENTS FOR HELPING TO CONCEAL AND ENHANCE THE RIGHT BITS, ESPECIALLY WHERE OUR MIDDLE IS CONCERNED. That's why it is worth investing in at least one for winter and one for summer.

I love to wear tailored jackets with jeans and skirts. It brings just the right amount of structure to an outfit. I find it much harder to wear little chiffon dresses. Skimpy things are tricky for me, and a lot of us. Tailored jackets rather than loose, unstructured jackets are fantastic for us as we age. They work with jeans, trousers, pencil skirts, full skirts and just about anything apart from hot pants, and we're not likely to be aiming for that as a look, are we, girls! A great jacket is one of the best investments you can make.

COATS

APART FROM BOOTS AND SHOES, MY NEXT FAVOURITE ITEM OF CLOTHING IS THE COAT. AS WE MOSTLY LIVE IN A COOLISH OR COLD CLIMATE, THE COAT IS A MUST FOR YOUR WARDROBE. Coats can be wonderfully flattering as well as providing you with warmth and coverage. Fitted coats are such a great way to look like you mean business. There are so many different styles of coat that I love. Military-inspired coats can be so chic on any age. They work with flat boots and skirts, trousers, just about anything (you can hide a lot underneath them too!).

If you pick the right coat, it can stay in fashion for years, e.g. the camel-hair wrap-around trench coat with tied belt and big collar – very Lauren Bacall and very sophisticated. A **BURBERRY** mackintosh cinched in at the waist is another classic style that works so well with a pencil skirt underneath, or unbuttoned and teamed with jeans for more casual outings. Big collars are wonderfully flattering and I love the way a frock coat can double up as a smart evening outfit. Team with big earrings, a clutch purse and very opaque tights, et *voilà*!

in the middle

184

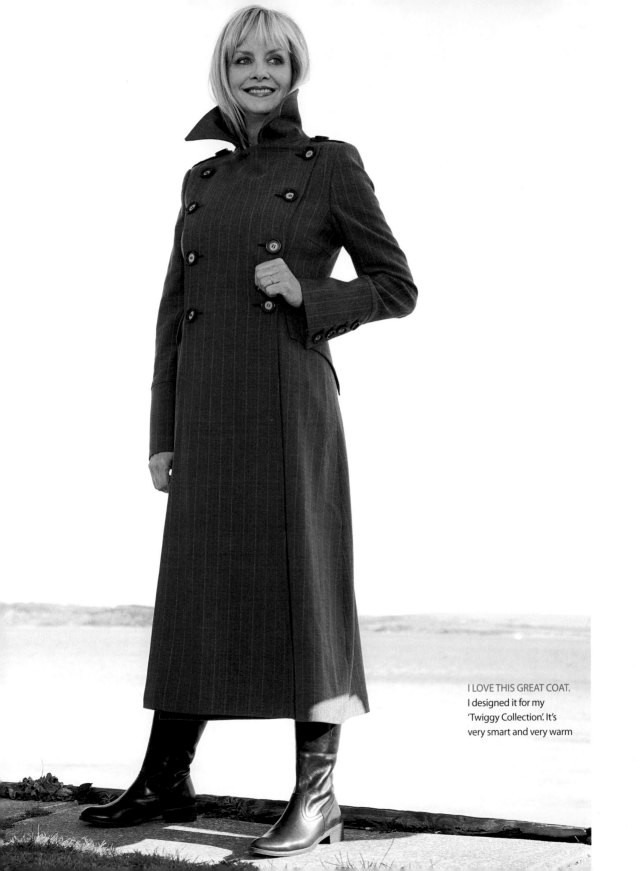

I LOVE THIS GREAT COAT.
I designed it for my
'Twiggy Collection'. It's
very smart and very warm

healthy *& fit*

WHEN WALLIS SIMPSON SAID YOU CAN NEVER BE TOO RICH OR TOO THIN, HOW WRONG SHE WAS! AS FOR BEING TOO RICH, WELL, THAT'S UP FOR DEBATE! But in my opinion you can certainly be too thin, which might sound funny coming from me. If I was as thin now as I was back when I was a teenager, I'd look gaunt. From middle age onwards, being too thin can be seriously ageing. Having said that, I don't know a single woman who hasn't put on some weight around her middle. It just happens and the key is to keep it in check. Exercise and diet are vital components in keeping healthy and fit. Whether you choose swimming, cycling, tennis, roller blading, even tap dancing, anything that gets the blood pumping is great. Try to do just twenty minutes a day and you will be amazed by the difference. Here are some of my suggestions for looking after yourself:

LONG WALKS

WE ALL KNOW WE SHOULD EXERCISE MORE, BUT SOMETIMES IT'S HARD TO FIT IT INTO OUR BUSY SCHEDULES. Don't despair. Walking is fab for you, so try to walk somewhere at least once a day. And I don't mean a gentle stroll. I'm talking about a brisk

186

stepping out. You might even work up a sweat! That's good. A couple of times a week, instead of jumping in the car or catching the bus, try walking the distance. It really works. If I'm in London, we always have a Sunday morning walk through the parks, often stopping off for brunch. In the countryside a long walk is a must on many levels.

Like all forms of exercise, it's not only your body that reaps the benefits. It's your mind and soul too. The wonderful thing about walking is that you can start to appreciate things you might otherwise not notice. Walking allows your mind to wander. It's a wonderful way of clearing the head. No matter how long or short the walk, make sure you wear comfy shoes. In the summer I'll wear a good pair of trainers; in winter I'll wear walking boots with a bit of ankle support. Dust down those walking shoes and get strolling!

POWER PLATE

I WENT TO MY FIRST POWER-PLATE CLASS: WHAT A FABULOUS EXPERIENCE. I was a bit nervous to start, but I really enjoyed it. It really worked my muscles. Each session is only twenty-five minutes, and you work through a series of exercises on the plate, which vibrates. It is a peculiar feeling, but not unpleasant (a bit like a high-powered version of a massage chair).

The beauty of Power Plate is, if you are working, you can go in your lunch hour. They advise two sessions a week, and I'm really looking forward to my next session. It supposedly tones up all the muscles and works on cellulite. A lot of A-list celebrities love it.

At the end of the session you lie in various positions, and it massages – very good for circulation. Just be warned, my muscles were a bit tight the day after (a bit like the soreness after a good session in the gym), but that proves my muscles had a workout.

To find a Power Plate studio near you, go to **http://uk.powerplate.com**

in the middle

187

PILATES

I HAVE ALWAYS DONE SOME FORM OF EXERCISE AND USED TO REGULARLY VISIT A GYM. But then I discovered Pilates, which is gentler and yet still works on the whole body. It can strengthen and lengthen your muscles, get rid of 'love handles' and release tension. And it can dramatically improve your posture, which can work wonders as we age. It is crucial to keep reminding yourself every day to have good posture. How often have you been sitting at a desk and become aware of your slouching position?

Originally developed in the early twentieth century by Joseph Pilates as a form of rehabilitation for injured soldiers and, later, dancers, Pilates has become extremely popular over the last decade and there are now studios nationwide. As Joseph Pilates himself said: 'Physical fitness is the first requisite of happiness. In order to achieve happiness, it is imperative to gain mastery of your body. If at the age of thirty you are stiff and out of shape, you are old. If at sixty you are supple and strong, then you are young.'

Due to imperfect posture, I have a weak lower back and need to strengthen my inner core to support it. Whenever I'm working abroad, I have thirty minutes of stretches which I can do anywhere. But sometimes the discipline of Pilates or any exercise is easier to do at a studio. Two sessions a week with a good teacher will be one of the best investments in your health and well-being. Once you get the hang of it, it will change your posture, improve your body shape, develop your strength and work wonders on the pelvic-floor muscles. I have a wonderful Pilates teacher, Dreas, and he has helped me enormously with my posture and getting strong. *(See the directory for details)*

If you would like to try it out, find your nearest instructor on the UK websites **www.pilatesfoundation.com** and **www.pilates.co.uk**. For the more adventurous and supple, there are many Pilates hybrids available too. One of these is **HEARTCOREPILATES**, which can be tried at a London-based studio using specially developed machines and a constantly moving routine. There is also **TENPILATES**, which many of my friends say has transformed their physique and relieved their back pain. But with anything more

in the middle

188

cardiovascular, consult your GP first and be sure to do only the movements that your body is comfortable with, to avoid risk of injury. **ALEXANDER TECHNIQUE** is another way to become more aware of your body and how it holds itself. Find a qualified teacher near you and see what a difference a few sessions make.

DANCING

MY FAVOURITE FORM OF EXERCISE IS TAP DANCING, WHICH I STARTED AT THE AGE OF TWENTY. It's great fun, works the whole body and the brain and you end up feeling like Fred Astaire! How wonderful. I still do my classes with my lovely teacher Ali Golding and love every minute. There are endless forms of dance, from salsa to ballroom. Google your area for your nearest dance studio and take the plunge – I promise that you'll love it.

MASSAGE

I LEARNED HOW BENEFICIAL A REGULAR MASSAGE CAN BE, NOT ONLY FOR YOUR BODY BUT ALSO FOR YOUR OVERALL WELL-BEING, when I was starring on Broadway in the musical *My One and Only*. Tap dancing in eight shows a week is really hard going and it was imperative to have a massage regularly. It really is preventative medicine and there's no doubt that regular massage from a trained therapist can help alleviate a wealth of problems and be healing in so many ways. For me, I find the best cure for back pain is massage and exercise. I know it can be expensive, but at the very least ask for a referral through your GP for physiotherapy. I try to make time for massage at least once a month, ideally more. I love a fantastic remedial massage, combined with reiki therapy, that London-based Janyce Welch does. Remedial massage works wonders at stretching out sore muscles and realigning the spine. If you really want to spoil yourself, give yourself a treat and go to a health farm or a spa break. To find a massage therapist near you, look at the following websites: **www.gcmt.org.uk** and **www.massagetherapy.co.uk**.

in the middle

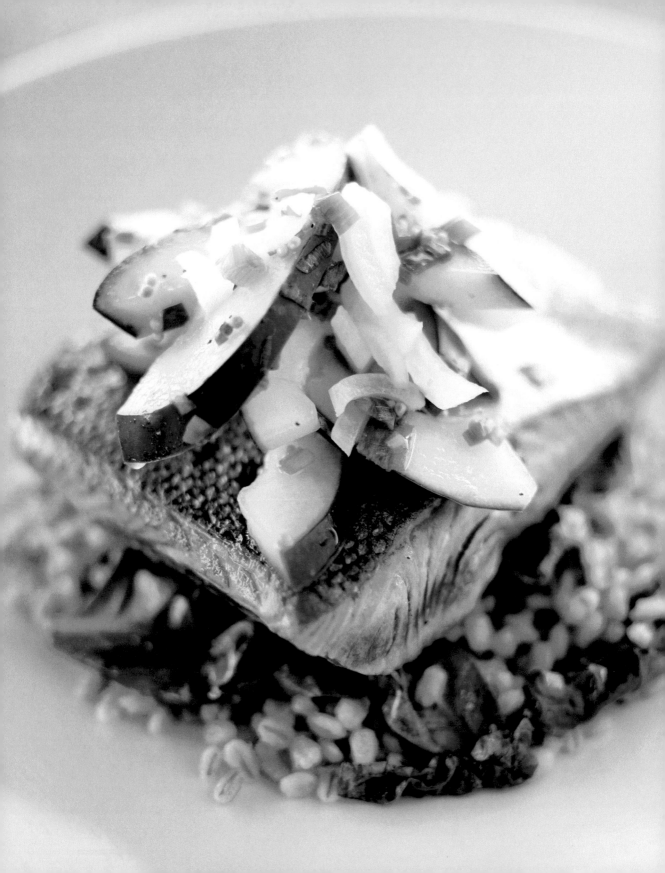

YOU ARE WHAT YOU EAT

I TRULY BELIEVE THE SAYING 'YOU ARE WHAT YOU EAT'. BY EATING HEALTHILY AND FOR SUSTENANCE, THERE'S NO NEED TO FOLLOW DIETS UNLESS YOU HAVE A SIGNIFICANT WEIGHT PROBLEM. Even then, the best way to lose weight is to exercise and cut down on portions. Think of ageing as ripening. What I mean is, don't get obsessive about being stick-thin. After all, not everyone is destined to be skinny. Instead, aim to be healthy and fit. Visit your GP and find out what your healthy weight should be. Chances are, you already know. Beware of crash diets. They are dangerous and do nothing except up-tip your metabolism. I've always been sceptical of 'fat free'. 'Fat free' can still mean packed full of sugar. Don't be deceived by it all, girls!

For me, eating well is all about re-learning a tasty and healthy way of eating. I choose organic whenever I can get it and always try to eat seasonal, local produce. Become obsessed with food in the right way. I used to love, love, love fish and chips. Suddenly, in my early fifties, I found it gave me terrible indigestion, which fried food in general does. Cheese and pickled onions are the same. I still love pickled onions but eat them sparingly. Cheese is fine, so long as it's not too close to bedtime. You have to get to know your body and work with it. Don't fight the inevitable, just support its changes with common sense.

The Mediterranean diet is so delicious. With its high content of fish, olive oil, fresh veg, high fibre and herbs, to me it makes nutritional sense too. I never cook in butter or use fat, apart from bacon. If I eat bacon I always grill it. I love butter on bread but if it's on my vegetables I hate it. It turns my stomach. It's too rich for me. I'd rather drizzle a bit of olive oil and salt or, even better, lemon juice and black pepper. I know it's bad for you but I love salt. Nobody's perfect! I'm not a huge vitamin-taker either. I've always had the philosophy that so long as you eat the right foods you'll get the good stuff. Fresh is best and a great investment is a juicer, although washing them is such a pain in the you-know-what. I have to admit that mine is in the cupboard gathering dust.

in the middle

191

It's not a sin to have a biscuit every now and then, but, as I keep saying, moderation is the key

Through my obsession with good food, I've become a very happy cook. I love experimenting with different ingredients and believe that buying organic and seasonal produce is really important. Cooking is good for the soul!

I do like to have a glass of wine or two with dinner, but not more. If I drink more than that, which happens occasionally, it makes me feel rotten. I was thrilled when I read that a glass or two of red wine is actually very good for you. It's full of antioxidants. Moderation in everything is a good yardstick, so long as you're not a party-pooper. The odd treat is good for the soul. If I fancy a piece of chocolate, I don't eat a whole bar in one gollop, instead I'll have a chunk or two and that does it. Dark chocolate is fine in small amounts and the best is **GREEN & BLACK'S** organic chocolate. I keep a bar on the top shelf of the fridge for quiet nibbles.

Although I very rarely have puddings after meals, in the winter I love home-made rice pudding, but not every night! My home-made apple and blackberry pie is another favourite. I make it without much sugar. It keeps it nice and tart. I'll serve it with custard, or you could replace the custard with vanilla yoghurt. You just have to be a bit disciplined with yourself. Snacking is a big vice. The packet of crisps, the biscuits with your tea, the chocolate bar or two in the afternoon. A Mars at eleven, two Milky Ways in the afternoon – that's crazy! Fizzy drinks aren't great either. If you're feeling peckish in between meals, have a glass of water, a cup of herbal tea and a piece of fruit, or a handful of nuts and raisins. Instead of a choccy biscuit, have a cracker with a little butter and Marmite or honey.

PORTIONS

LOTS OF PEOPLE ARE GIVEN A PLATE OF FOOD AND WANT TO FINISH IT ALL. IF I HAVE A PLATE OF FOOD, I EAT UNTIL I'M FULL AND THEN I STOP. A good way to guide your portions is to hold out your hands in front of you, palms facing upwards and cupped together in a bowl shape. In one palm, that's the amount of protein to have per meal. In the other is the amount of carbohydrate or starch. Both hands cupped together show the amount of veg/fruit to have at the same meal. This portion system is much more realistic and true to your own body size.

AND FINALLY ... A WORD ABOUT MEAT

I'M NOT A BIG MEAT EATER. I LOVE CHICKEN AND FISH AND OCCASIONALLY RED MEAT, BUT I ONLY EVER BUY ORGANIC. Meat tastes better when organic. I instinctively feel it is not wise to eat meat that has been pumped full of antibiotics. Animal welfare is also incredibly important to me. Battery farming is so abhorrent it should be banned.

The problem is that organic meat is pricier. But it has been proven that too much red meat, particularly, is bad for you. Cut down on your meat intake and save the pennies for a delicious once-a-week organic treat. Substitute meat with oily fish, grilled or baked, at least twice a week. Sardines are so good for you and don't cost much at all. I love herring too. I recently bought five herrings at a fishmonger's near to me in the country and he charged me one pound. Now that's what I call a bargain, and so delicious!

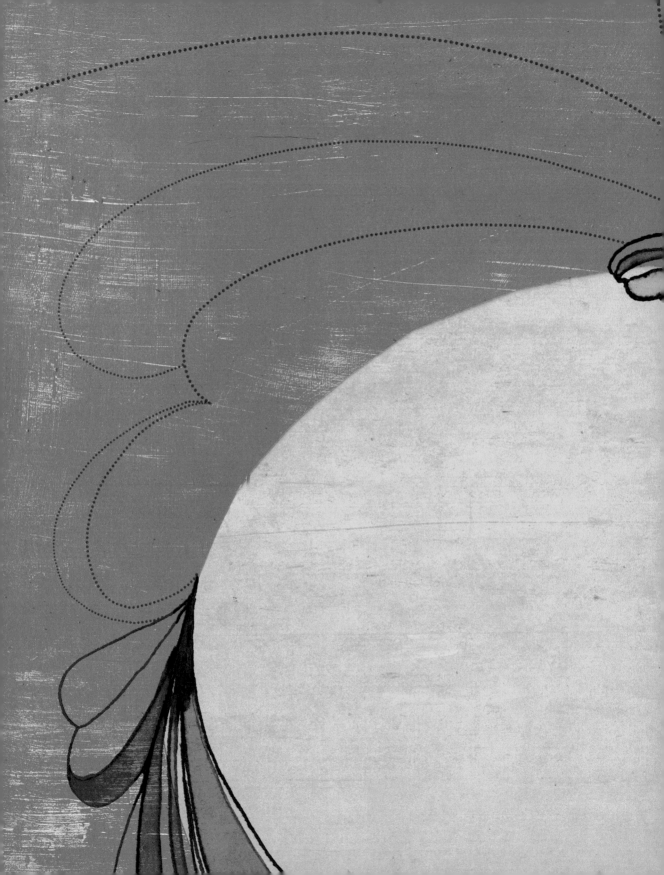

chapter six
*dressing
down*

I NEVER REALLY THINK ABOUT WHAT KIND OF STYLE I HAVE. I'M OBSESSED BY CLOTHES, BUT I DON'T THINK I HAVE A PARTICULAR STYLE. I DON'T CONSIDER MYSELF AS HIGHLY ELEGANT AND SOPHISTICATED. MY STYLE IS KIND OF CASUAL, COMFORTABLE – I LOVE TO BE COMFORTABLE, WHICH IS WHY I LIKE MEN'S SUITS – AND ECLECTIC.

There's a little bit of boho in my wardrobe choices too. One thing I must confess to loving, and I'm proud to come out of the closet with this . . . is tracksuits. Thankfully, we've come a long way since elasticated trousers. My mum swore by them, and a lot of older women do, simply for the comfort factor. But let's face it, tracksuits are for indoors or the gym only. Most people look dreadful in them, myself included, but I love lounging around in mine at home. I put on a tracksuit as soon as I'm through the front door. I call them my comfies. I take everything off except my knickers, then put on a big sweatshirt top and unmatching tracksuit bottoms. I'm not a fashion icon at home! And I don't care a hoot that the world is so divided on whether or not they are fashionable. For the ultimate in foot comfort, you cannot beat Ugg boots. I have worn mine for the last fifteen years. They are a great alternative to wellies on a walk and there's nothing like them for keeping feet snug, whether pottering around at home, or dashing out. I think they look great too.

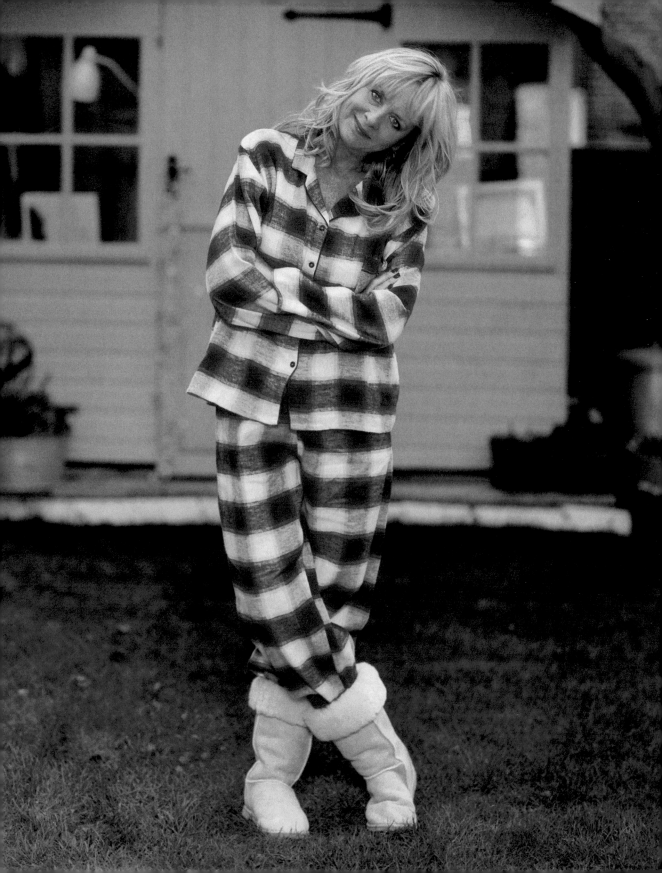

FOR PASHMINAS YOU MIGHT LIKE TO TRY

- *PURE COLLECTION – offer classics like the Pashmina Shawl. Available in a beautiful array of colours from honeysuckle to mulberry.*
- *BRORA – not technically a pashmina, but Brora do sumptuously soft cashmere stoles and shawls. The lacy wrap is a classic.*

Cosy clothes that look and feel like a treat, rather than a sloppy afterthought, are available somewhere out there; you just have to know where to look. It's the same with pyjamas, dressing gowns, slippers and all the things we sleep in and wear on lazy Sundays.

It's well worth investing in a couple of cashmere sweaters and chunky cardigans. Cashmere wrap cardigans are very kind to all shapes and sizes. Layer them over a crisp white shirt, or with a T-shirt on weekends, and you can team this with jeans, a skirt or trousers. There is something so luxurious about cashmere and not only is it readily available on the high street these days, it is also much cheaper than it used to be. You could also look out for merino wool and cotton jersey, if your budget prefers.

Another cosy favourite is a pashmina. These hide a lot of ills if you drape them carefully, and come in such gorgeous colours. In the warmer months they come in handy to drape over the shoulders as a shawl.

Pashminas keep you warm in winter and are a great alternative to cosy cardigans

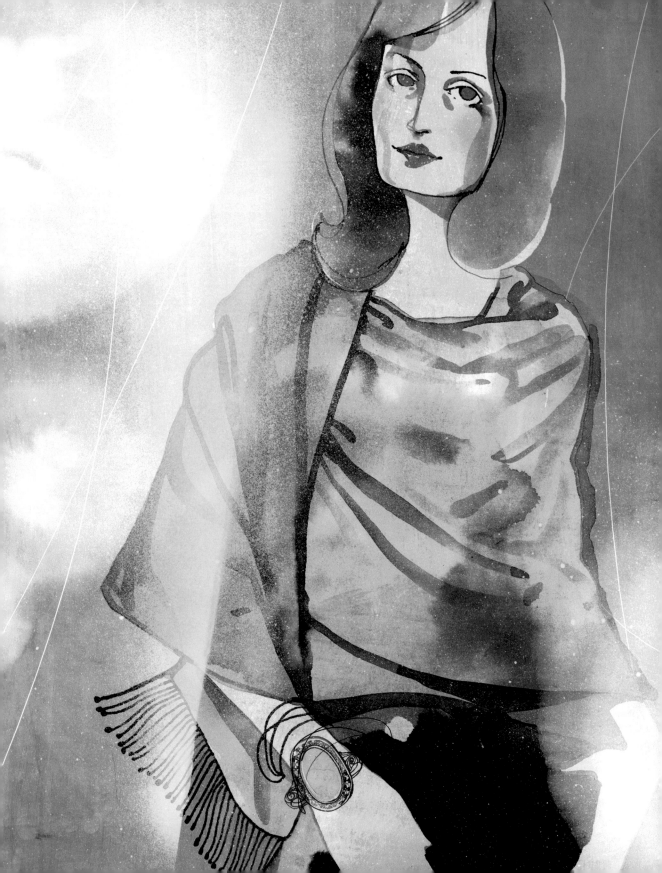

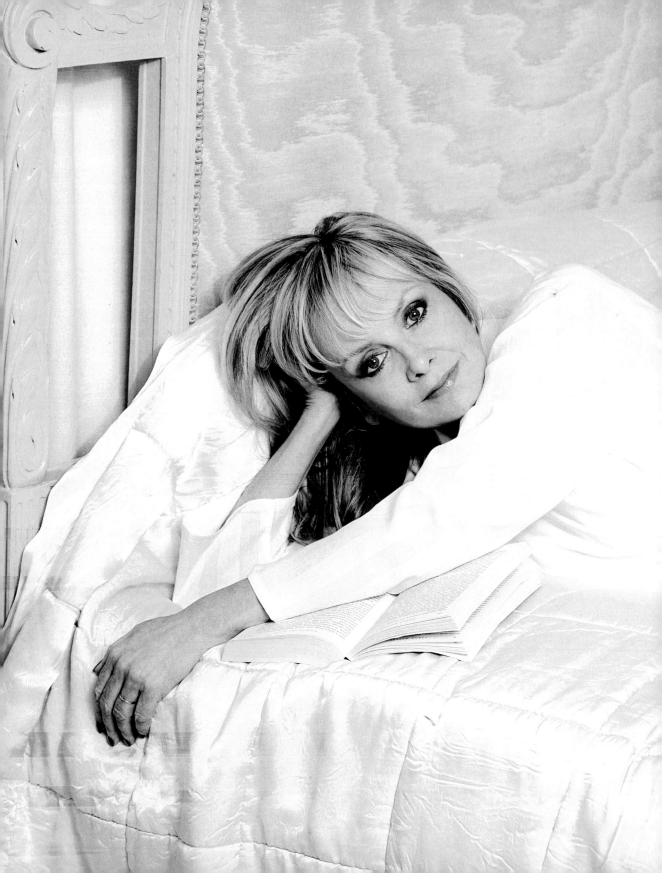

Great *dressing-down* shops to try . . .

- **SWEATY BETTY** – Their range is Cool Gym. Look out for the wrap tops (wear loosely tied round the hips, or tied ballet-style round the waist). Very feminine, and flatters the figure really well.

- **THE WHITE COMPANY** – Lovely natural-fabric basics are repeated each season. A great place for lounge-wear. Look out for the cashmere trousers and jersey cotton-mix wrap tops and trousers.

- **SPLENDID** – Although pricey, **SPLENDID,** a label from America, makes the best T-shirts, tracksuits and cotton dresses.

- **TOAST** – Gorgeous drawstring trousers in pretty colours, and the best pyjamas and dressing gowns in the world.

- **M&S** – The soft Velour Drawstring Joggers and Velour String Tie Hooded Jacket are bestsellers. Also has gorgeous cashmere joggers.

- **HUSH** – This mail-order-only range produces luxuriously comfortable loungewear. Their Knitted Lounge Pants, Sloppy Jumper and full-length Cardigown are brilliant.

- **BRORA** – Does lovely cashmere tweed trousers and soft, striped crew-neck sweaters, perfect for country walks and cosy weekends at home. Their cardigans are an all-year investment staple (check out their website for sale bargains).

dressing down

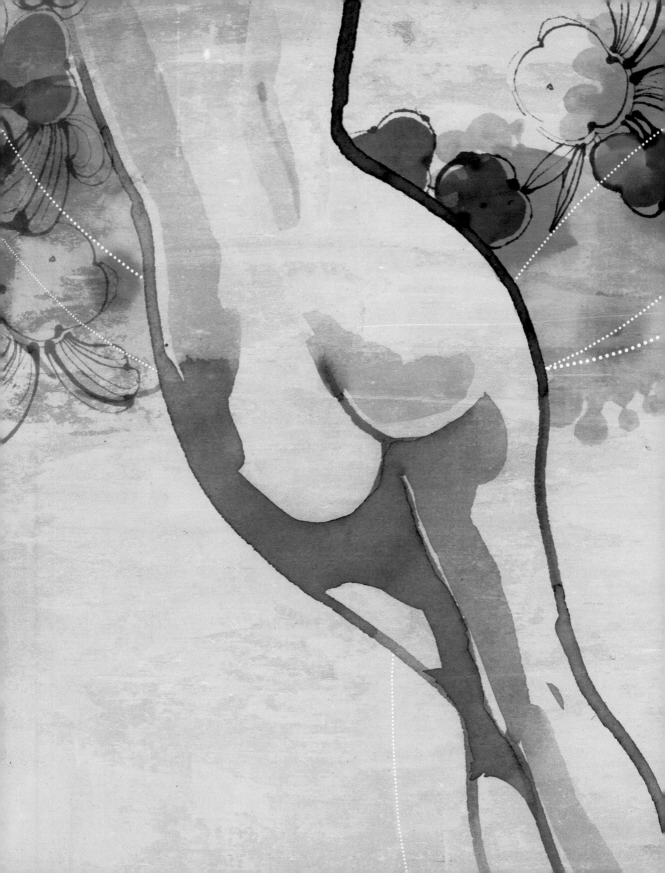

bums & hips

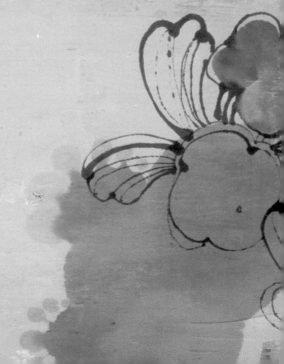

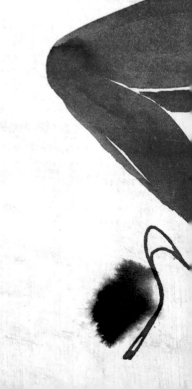

I'VE ALWAYS HAD A BOYISH FIGURE. NO WAIST, JUST STRAIGHT UP AND DOWN. AS WE GET OLDER, DEPENDING ON OUR NATURAL BODY SHAPE, ONE OF TWO THINGS USUALLY HAPPENS: EITHER WE DEVELOP BIGGER BOTTOMS, OR, IN SLIM WOMEN, THE BOTTOM BECOMES FLAT. As well as that, I'm afraid to say, just like our boobs, the bum can droop too. You might also discover you have cellulite and stretch marks.

One of the best ways to prevent this is healthy eating combined with regular exercise. I have already mentioned Pilates, but on its own this does not burn fat, so include more cardio by power-walking every day or finding an exercise routine that suits you.

bums & hips

204

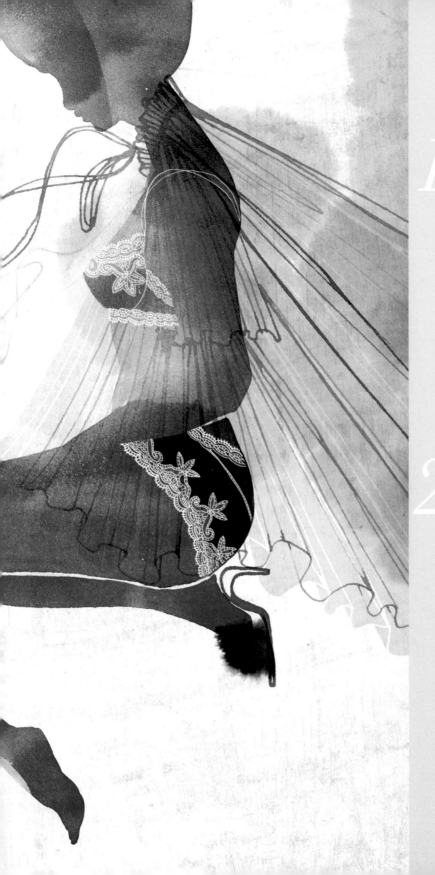

CREAMS
YOU MIGHT
LIKE TO TRY

1

Cellulite Creams

LUXURY

- *Clarins Body Shaping Supplement*

MIDDLE

- *Environ Body Sculpt Gel*

BUDGET

- *L'Oréal Paris Perfect Slim Pro Massage*

2

Body Creams

LUXURY

- *Lancôme Nutrix Royal Body*

MIDDLE

- *Dermalogica Body Hydrating Cream*

BUDGET

Revlon Dry Skin Relief

ON THE KNICKER LINE

Wherever possible, you should try to match your bra colour to your knickers

VERY PLEASANT LADIES MUST NEVER HAVE VPLS BUT IT AMAZES ME HOW MANY YOU SEE OUT THERE. IS THE REASON A HEALTHY LACK OF VANITY? I've come to the conclusion that many women just don't check their rear view once they've got dressed, and this is where the VPL can sneak up on the chicest of suspects.

If your knickers are too tight, they will create bumps, so it really is best to ditch them. I have never been a fan of thongs; they are best described as floss for the derrière. Do I want to be uncomfortable? No thanks! There are plenty of knicker shapes available and it's over to you to find ones that are comfortable and fit properly. My favourites for everyday wear are hi-leg knickers. They're so comfy. If you're wearing figure-hugging dresses and trousers, it's a great idea to invest in tummy flatteners *(see the section on waists and tums in Chapter Five)*. Not only do they help hold it all in, they also create a smooth line under whatever you're wearing. I have size 10 and size 12 pairs and fluctuate between the two. They can be just as successful holding in the behind as the front! Whatever size you are, they are a must under tight skinny dresses or skirts.

Believe it or not, a lot of us don't bother wearing matching underwear. It's a small thing, but makes us feel good knowing that what lurks beneath is all in order. Having said that, if you want to wear your best white bra with a giant pair of pink frilly knickers, be my guest!

You can buy great <u>knickers</u> at . . .

- <u>**M&S**</u> – The **SHAPEWEAR** range of lingerie is perfect for sucking you in, in all the right places. Try the **LIGHT CONTROL UNDERWIRED MULTIWAY BODY**, an all-in-one that helps to keep a slim silhouette, whatever you're wearing. Similarly, the **MAGIC FIRM CONTROL WAIST CINCHER** cuts tummy bulge under dresses and skirts.

- <u>**SLOGGI**</u> – The **CONTROL MAXI BRIEF** is a high-waisted pair of briefs that gives good coverage and support but doesn't cut into your flesh.

- <u>**CALVIN KLEIN UNDERWEAR**</u> – The **PERFECTLY FIT SEDUCTION** range (balconette bra, low-rise shorts) is a new seam-free invention that fits nicely beneath tight-fitting clothing.

- <u>**ELLE MACPHERSON INTIMATES**</u> – The **SKIN LIGHTS** range is a microfine lingerie range with no hard lines.

- <u>**HANRO**</u> – Their range of laser-cut knickers that disappear under clothes uses sheer mercerized cotton for a comfortable and close fit.

- <u>**COMMANDO**</u> – Invisible under virtually anything, these knickers are low-risers and lie completely flat against the skin. They contain no elastic and have no trim.

- <u>**BODAS**</u> – They make some of the best-cut hipster briefs. They won't leave you with unseemly lines beneath your trousers as they are cut just below the bottom cheek. The fabrics are microfine to prevent any lumps and bumps under clothing. Try the **SHEER MESH FRENCH KNICKERS**, or the **COTTON BASICS HIPSTER BRIEF**.

- <u>**STELLA MCCARTNEY**</u> – New range of pretty undies in gorgeous fabrics. I just love her 'Days of the Week' knickers. Quite expensive but lovely.

bums & hips

207

jeans

JEANS FORM A HUGE PART OF MY WARDROBE. I LOVE MY JEANS. I HAVE THEM IN ALL DIFFERENT COLOURS, STYLES AND SHAPES. IF THERE'S ONE THING I AM LIKELY TO PICK UP EVERY COUPLE OF SEASONS, IT'S A NEW PAIR. In recent years, the denim market has become saturated with high-end, luxury denim labels. The high street has gone crazy for denim too, with stretchy, boot-cut, hipster, high-waist, wide-leg, capri, boyfriend, bumster, tumster, marble-wash, indigo and ever-varying shapes, colours and cuts available in almost every size.

What this choice means is that there is every possibility you can find the perfect pair of jeans to suit your body shape. However, it can be a daunting challenge to seek out the perfect pair. Set plenty of time aside for buying jeans. It's worth doing the research and trying on as many as you can, as I guarantee you will eventually luck out.

For older women, it is a great fortune that hipster denim is no longer the sole cut available. Hipster cuts are not kind to anybody with a belly. All they do is accentuate the bulge. Worse still, just like one of my girlfriends who has had two C-sections, you'll end up with loose tum overspill flopping on top of the belt loops and have people asking if you're pregnant again. One of my friends swears by maternity jeans for comfort. Some of the higher-end labels have the best-quality denim plus a supremely comfy tummy panel. So long as you wear tops that cover to the hip bone, who's going to know? Hipsters also have the propensity to flash your pants and more to the world when you bend over. Not a good look, and hardly dignified for us damsels.

bums & hips

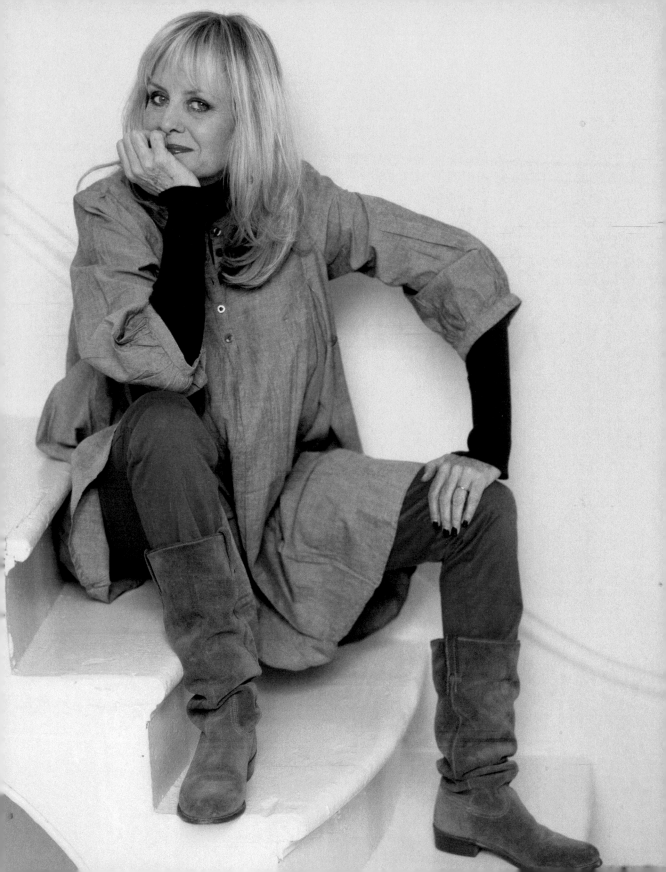

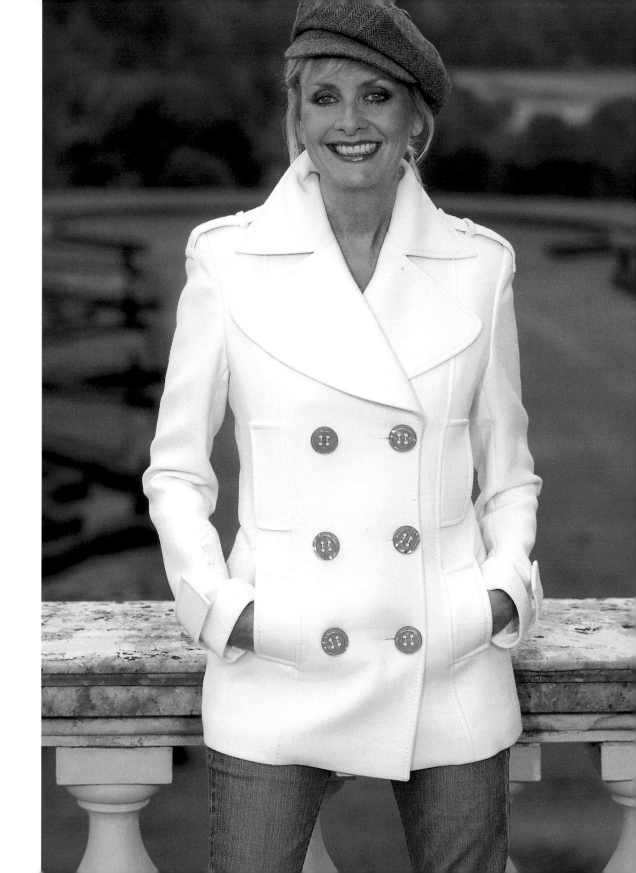

I have loved skinny jeans since the eighties. When I was much younger, my skinny legs were a joke, really. I certainly got teased about them as a teenager, but I have always worn tight jeans to accentuate them. In the eighties, I went through a major skin-tight denim phase. I loved Fiorucci and lived in a pair of shiny maroon spray-on jeans. I also had a great emerald-green pair and some black satin ones. I used to wear them with flat ankle boots and a top with big padded shoulders. No sniggering, girls, it's a look that's coming round again. Just you wait!

I love corduroy jeans as well as vertical-striped jeans. Both are a fun switch from plain old denim. They can be slimming so long as the stripes aren't too chunky. Until the skinny jeans became readily available a few years ago, I always wore boot-cut jeans. For older, more slender women, 'boyfriend' jeans, or men's jeans cut for women, are a truly comfortable style. They're not huge, but they're baggy in the front so I pull them in with a belt, slung a little low.

If you absolutely love the hipster shape, consider teaming them with big sweaters to cover the waistband, or layer them with long T-shirts that cover the hips and dreaded 'muffin top' haunches. There's no question, denim is here to stay!

Tailored jackets with jeans is a great look for all ages. Dress up with a heel and a pretty shirt, or just wear a smart T-shirt under the jacket. It's a great look for daytime

You might like to try these <u>Tips</u> before you hit the pavements in search of your dream pair . . .

1 **JEANS RULE NUMBER ONE:** you have to try them on. Never assume they will fit you. Just like underwear, jeans manufacturers have their own sizing system, so make sure they are the right size. If you don't trust yourself, take a friend whose opinion you value and don't feel shy about pestering the staff.

2 **IF YOU THINK YOU HAVE FOUND A GREAT PAIR,** put them on hold while you research other options. That way, you know you can go back to them at the end of your research.

3 **LONG JEANS CAN MAKE LEGS LOOK LONGER AND SLIMMER,** especially if you wear them with heels.

4 **AVOID WEARING JEANS WITH LOW, POINTY, KITTEN HEELS AT ALL COSTS,** as this can make you look top-heavy.

5 **HIGH-WAISTED JEANS ARE READILY AVAILABLE** and a great alternative to hipsters. If you have a protruding tummy, cover/layer the waistband area with a sweater, longer jacket or shirt.

6 **THE POSITIONING OF THE POCKETS ON THE BEHIND CAN MAKE SUCH A DIFFERENCE TO YOUR BOTTOM.** Denim designer Paige Adams-Geller, the fit model for many of the high-end, LA-based denim labels, whose own label I love, suggests your bottom should look like two ripe, juicy cherries.

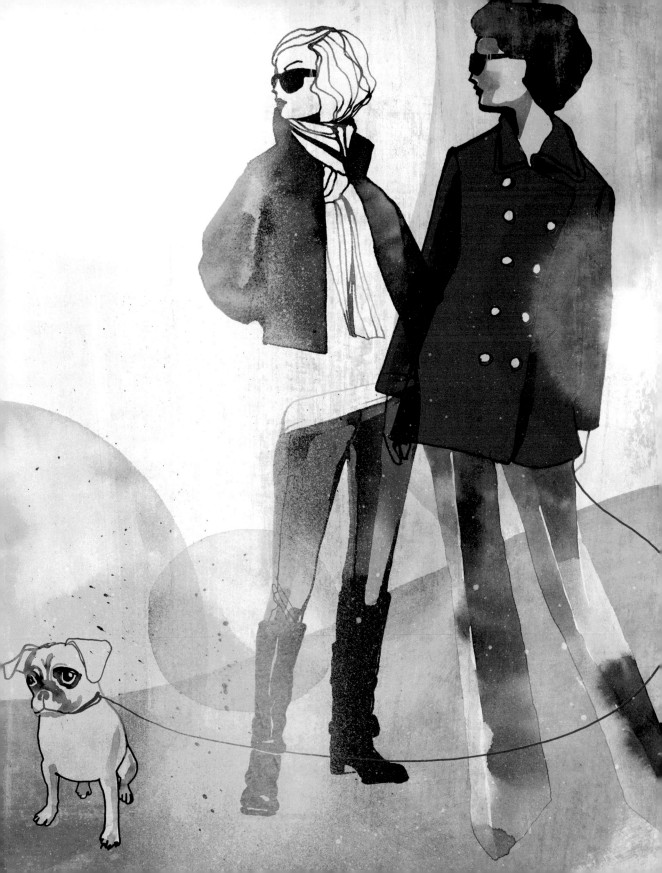

Hot _denim_ to try

Don't be bullied into spending more on a pair of jeans than you want or have to

- **GAP** – For all shapes and cuts, it's a great place to start. I love their skinny jeans as they have enough stretch to make them super-comfy.

- **EVANS** – Offers a comprehensive range of styles, including straight-leg, boot-cut, wide-leg and cropped jeans. Sizes from 14 to 32. Their website offers a section called _'Find your perfect fit'_, which offers outfit suggestions and helpful advice on finding denim for your body shape.

- **DOROTHY PERKINS** – Offers a good range of skinny, boot-cut and straight-leg styles. Sizes from 6 to 22.

- **WAREHOUSE** – Their **70S WIDE LEG JEAN** in dark denim and the **AGED KICK FLARE** look great with a heel or chunky boot and really add length to your legs.

- **UNIQLO** – Super value and brilliant-fitting slim jeans. Adequate for most shapes, they have just the right amount of stretch, and the price means you can buy two for the price of one! Try their skinny-fit straight jeans or boot-cut-fit jeans.

- **KAREN MILLEN** – Does a good range of denim; opt for boot-cut or straight-leg styles over skinnies.

- **FREEMANS** – Stocks a good range of classic denim labels like **LEE**, **WRANGLER** and **LEVIS**. Sometimes it's worth experimenting at home, where you can try on many different styles and find what you like best. Ordering from a multi-brand mail-order catalogue enables you to get great brands at competitive prices, and free returns.

- <u>**LITTLEWOODS DIRECT**</u> – Stocks a good range of jeans.

- <u>**SEVEN FOR ALL MANKIND**</u> – Higher end of the price range, but classic shapes they keep doing from season to season. When they fit, they fit you perfectly, plus their maternity jeans are great for comfort.

- <u>**PAIGE PREMIUM DENIM**</u> – Great for all ages but super-flattering for older women as they hug and enhance the figure, rather than cut into it. **THE BENEDICT CANYON SLIM BOOTCUT JEAN** has a slight kick flare and is cut slim on the leg, making your legs look long and elegant. You can even check out the **PAIGE DENIM** online interactive fit guide.

- <u>**NYDJ**</u> – The infamous **TUMMY TUCK JEAN** does as it says on the packet and keeps everything nicely cinched in round the waist. They contain 4 per cent Lycra so it is advisable to buy them one size down from your regular size.

- <u>**RALPH LAUREN**</u> – Brilliant straight-leg jeans in very dark denim.

- <u>**ARMANI JEANS**</u> – Not as expensive as a lot of the newer labels. Large range of classic shapes that come up a little higher on the waistline. Good for the tummy, and they make your bum look higher.

- <u>**HUDSON JEANS**</u> – Sexy, soft, casual denim, which is comfortable and easy to wear. Wide-leg and straight-leg styles are the best.

- <u>**TOAST**</u> – Dark, soft denim in simple styles that suit a womanly figure. Good price point.

- <u>**AMERICAN APPAREL**</u> – The best slim-fit, stretchy corduroy jeans on the market. A 65-year-old friend of mine, who has four grandchildren, has one in every colour and wears them with ankle boots and sweaters. A fab, gorgeous-granny look!

- <u>**MADE IN HEAVEN**</u> – A great Brit label that began in the seventies and stays true to its heritage. The **BERLIN** is a great high-waisted, bum-flattering style, while **PARIS** gently skims the ankle and looks great with flat pumps or loafers.

- <u>**WWW.DESIGNERDENIM.COM**</u> – A fabulous website stocking a huge range of designer denim in various styles, washes and price points – a great browsing tool when considering a denim purchase!

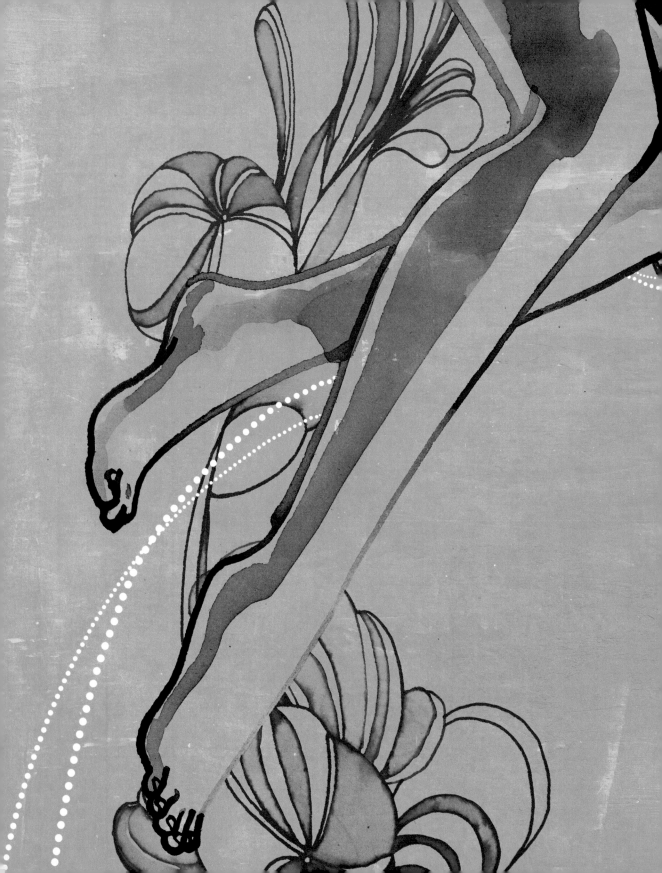

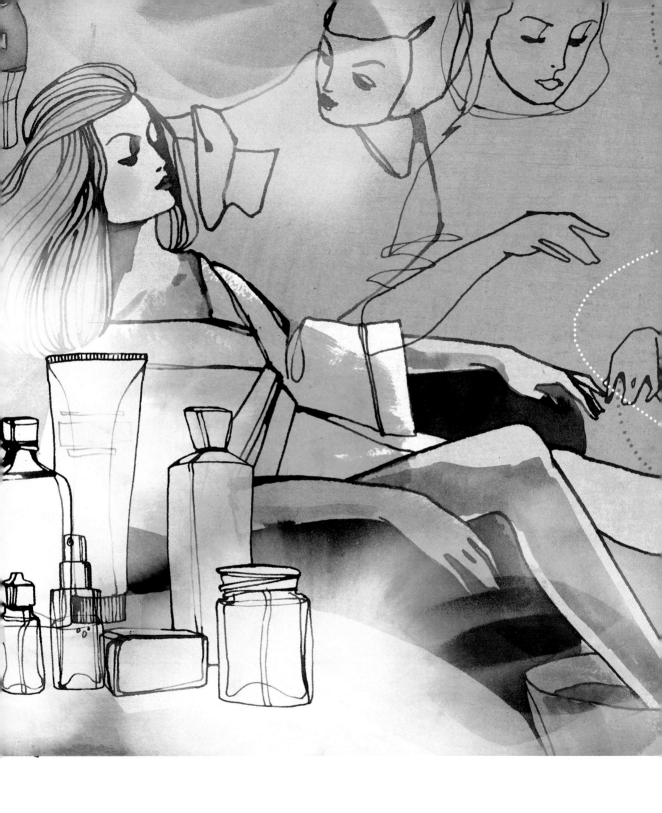

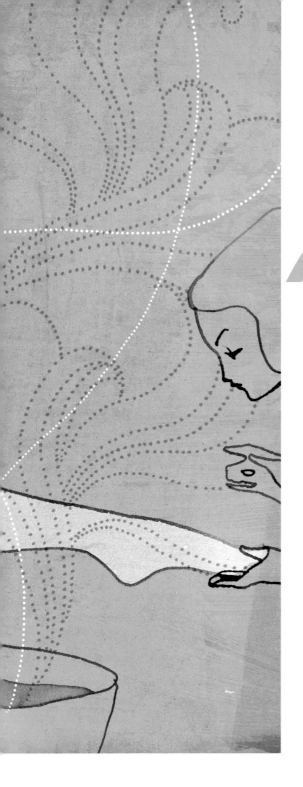

I DON'T MIND THE REST OF MY BODY NOT BEING BROWN, BUT IN THE SUMMER AND ON HOLIDAY I LOVE HAVING BROWN LEGS. NEVER UNDERESTIMATE THE POWER OF A WARM GLOW TO THE SKIN IN MAKING YOU LOOK AND FEEL GOOD.

For this purpose, unless you already have gorgeous, dark skin, fake tan is nothing less than fab. Used sparingly, it makes you feel so much better, so long as you choose the right shade and don't end up looking like a satsuma. And for heaven's sake, don't ever, ever do a sunbed. There should be no excuse! If DIY is too much to face, go and get airbrushed at your local beauty salon.

A few days before you head off on holiday is the time to apply fake tan. That way, your legs' first outing by the pool or on the beach won't be quite so scary. Softly tanned skin is kinder to wrinkles, lumps and bumps and those dreaded thread veins.

legs

219

skirts

GYPSY SKIRTS

HOORAY FOR THE GYPSY SKIRT. THERE ARE SO MANY VARIATIONS, THEY ARE SO FLATTERING AND YOU CAN HIDE A LOT UNDER THERE! You can wear them with a beautiful off-the-shoulder top, dress them down with a simple T-shirt, or up with belts and big sweaters in the winter. Invest in a gypsy skirt teamed with a skin-tight cashmere polo neck, and on any shape it looks gorgeous. It's sexy too. Men like it! I've hung on to my gypsy skirts as they never really seem to go out of fashion.

A great look has always been slouchy boots and gypsy skirts worn with scrunched-up velvet jackets and tight T-shirts underneath. I have velvet ones in winter and in summer they are great in floaty silks and soft cottons with a pair of jewelled sandals.

PENCIL SKIRTS

IF YOU'VE GOT THE BODY AND THE CHUTZPAH, A PENCIL SKIRT IS SO SEXY ON OLDER WOMEN. Look for ones that fall just below the knee, not above or on the knee. Think 1940s, cinched-in jackets, imagine you are Lauren Bacall on a date with Humphrey Bogart and you just absolutely have to wear very, very, very high heels – no excuses!

If I wear a tight skirt, those magic knickers help, or if you are too tummy-conscious, wear a pencil skirt, layer it with something that meets the top of the leg and throw on a big belt.

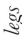
legs

220

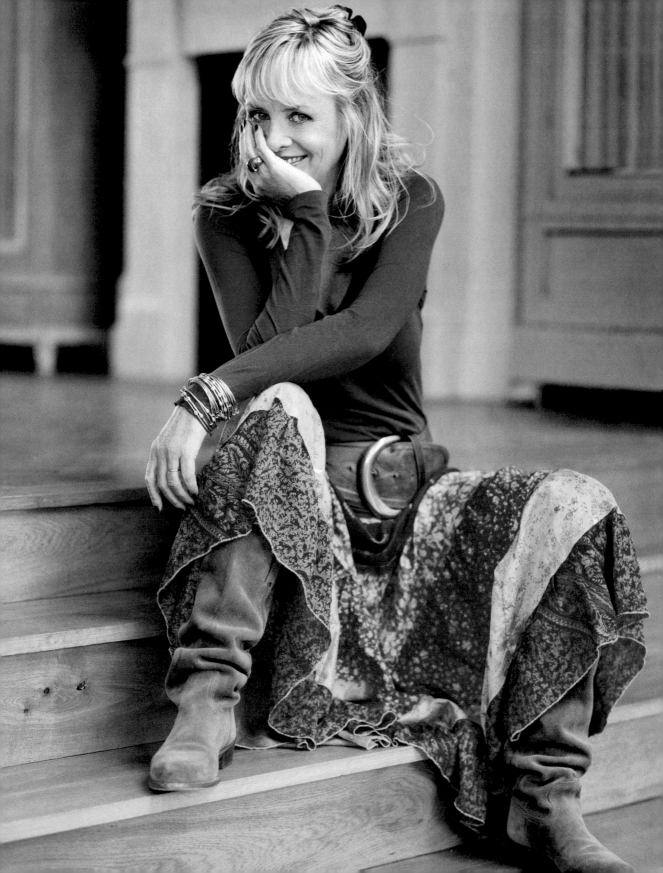

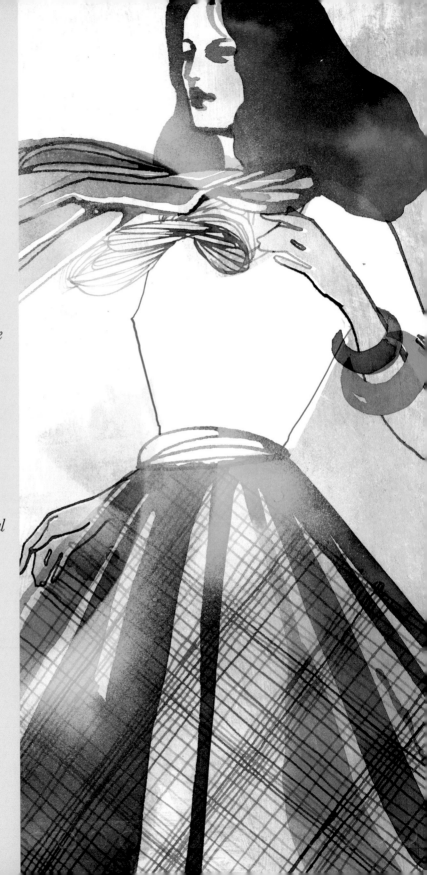

FOR SKIRTS
YOU MIGHT
LIKE TO TRY

- *WHISTLES – Good selection of tailored gabardine skirts for work.*
- *TOAST – Pleated skirts are flattering and versatile.*
- *HOBBS – Good selection of work and formal skirts.*
- *BODEN – Good for casual flippy A-line skirts, printed floral and plain silk skirts.*
- *L. K. BENNETT – Sharp fitted wool or linen tweed work skirts.*
- *JIGSAW – Delicate floral-print bias-cut skirts.*

FULL SKIRTS

I HAVE A FEW GATHERED KNEE-LENGTH SKIRTS WITH GIANT POCKETS. These are so flattering on, but can look like sacks on the clothes hanger. Dress them up with a white T-shirt, a scarf tied at the neck and a great bangle, and *voilà*! I also love pleated skirts and kilts. Kilts can be a great addition to your winter wardrobe. They look fabulous with a black polo neck, black tights and slouchy boots, and there are so many tartans to choose from.

MINISKIRTS

UNLESS YOU'VE GOT UNBELIEVABLY LONG, GORGEOUS LEGS, IT'S VERY HARD TO LOOK GOOD WEARING A MINISKIRT ONCE YOU REACH THE AGE OF FORTY, although you can wear a skirt a few inches above the knee if you team it with opaque tights. Instead, I would wear a tunic top with skin-tight jeans. And there you have the same sort of look, and I love it. In the winter, big sloppy jumpers that come to miniskirt length, with tight black jeans, a big belt and boots, is a chic way to reference that look, but you've got plenty of coverage and it's really comfy.

The key with this full-skirt shape is to balance it out with a great figure-hugging top

legs

223

tights

I'VE BEEN WEARING OPAQUE, BRIGHTLY COLOURED TIGHTS SINCE I WAS A TEENAGER. I ACTUALLY DID A RANGE OF TWIGGY TIGHTS IN THE SIXTIES – ALL OPAQUE BRIGHT COLOURS. In fact, I've never worn sheer stockings or hosiery. They don't work for me. If I want natural legs, I prefer fake tan. In the winter, there's nothing more fun than a black jumper and skirt with bright tights and black boots. Tights can really pull an outfit together. Avoid patterned tights. These are tricky to carry off and I always steer clear of them. Thick woolly tights are great for winter. They are so warm. Stockings can work, but they are so hard to wear outside of the bedroom. I have quite a collection of opaque tights. At the moment I've been wearing lots of purples, lavenders, fuchsias, sludgy jade, burgundy and chocolate brown. With certain things I do love plain black footless tights. I've also got a pair with lace around the bottom which can look lovely with ballet pumps. Make sure they are long enough. There's nothing more unflattering than leggings or footless tights that end halfway down the calf. If you're going to wear leggings, team them with a big shirt and a pair of flip-flops. This is a great look for summer.

Websites like **www.tightsplease.co.uk** and **www.mytights.com** are handy one-stop shops for all of our hoisery needs.

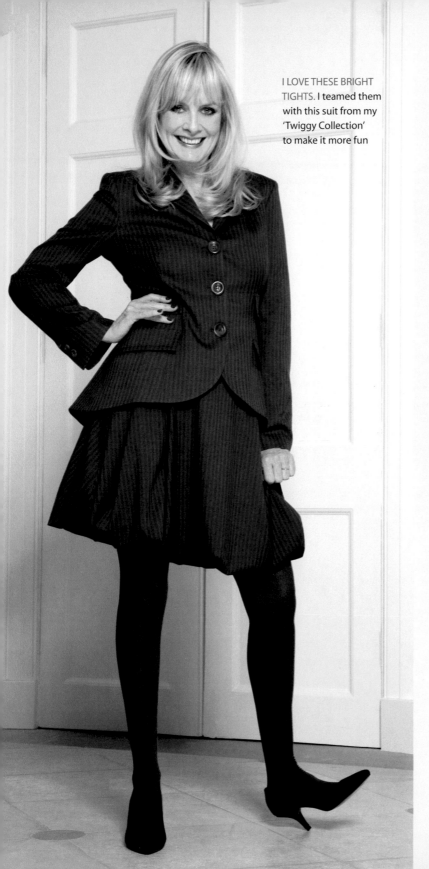

I LOVE THESE BRIGHT TIGHTS. I teamed them with this suit from my 'Twiggy Collection' to make it more fun

FOR TIGHTS
YOU MIGHT LIKE TO TRY

- *WOLFORD – the best-quality hosiery. They have the best black opaques – 'velvet de luxe' and 'satin opaques'.*
- *FALKE – does brilliant merino-wool tights for winter and also wool leggings, plus fine-wool long socks.*
- *M&S – has a good selection of tights at very reasonable prices (buy one size up as they tend to be tight round the waist).*
- *ARISTOC, CHARNOS AND PRETTY POLLY – are excellent for everyday tights and decent-quality black opaques too.*

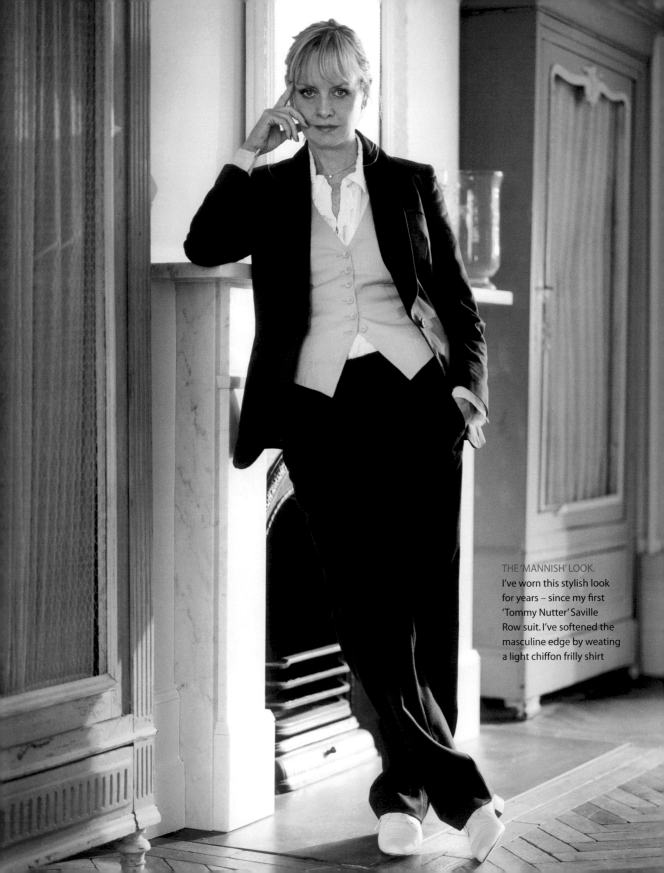

THE 'MANNISH' LOOK.
I've worn this stylish look
for years – since my first
'Tommy Nutter' Saville
Row suit. I've softened the
masculine edge by weating
a light chiffon frilly shirt

trousers

I AM REALLY A TROUSER GIRL, MUCH MORE THAN A DRESS GIRL. I'VE GOT SO MANY PAIRS AND SEEM TO BE ON A PERMANENT QUEST TO FIND THE PERFECT TROUSERS. Depending on the shape of your legs, trousers can be harder to wear than skirts, simply due to the fit. Everyone should have a pair of black tailored trousers that fit them well. **GAP** trousers are cut very boyish, which suits my shape. In winter I love big men's tweed trousers with a sweater and waistcoat. I love that look on women, but I do think you have to be on the slim side to carry it off well.

My two *top trouser* tips

1 **IF YOU FAVOUR HIGH-WAISTED TROUSERS** and have a bit of a tummy, you don't have to cover up the waist area completely. Instead, layer your look with a structured, tailored jacket or a cardigan.

2 **ANOTHER TUM FLATTENER WHEN WEARING TROUSERS** is to ensure you invest in tops that cover the crotch zone. A man's shirt can look chic. Roll up the sleeves and layer it with a long-sleeved T-shirt, leaving some of the top buttons open. This is much more flattering on a sticking-out tum. Pile on a few beads, and *voilà*!

legs

227

It may seem quite extravagant, but a couple of pairs of tailored trousers to suit your body shape can last a lifetime

PEDAL PUSHERS

CURVY GIRLS CAN LOOK AS FABULOUS IN PEDAL PUSHERS as slim girls, but shiny tanned legs are a must. Remember those fifties pin-ups? I love pedal pushers with a baggy top and a pair of heeled espadrilles in the summer. If you're short and curvy, team pedal pushers with a giant cinched-in belt over a to-the-hip cotton shirt or top. This can look great with flats for high summer. In fact, it's a fabulous look for all shapes and size.

CIGARETTE PANTS

I LOVE THIS SHAPE. THEY CAN LOOK GREAT ON ANY AGE OR FIGURE. 'Wear them with a short, sharp jacket or top and you'll look really modern, or a bigger-shaped, hip-length top and you'll still achieve a streamlined silhouette,' suggests Betty Jackson.

MEN'S TROUSERS

THE MAN'S SHAPE CAN WORK SO WELL, BUT IT'S WORTH INVESTING IN ALTERATIONS AT A GOOD DRY-CLEANER IF THERE'S ANY DISCREPANCY IN SIZE. If you find one pair too tight on the waist, but perfect on the leg, buy the next size up and have them taken in. Better still, visit a tailor and invest your pennies and pounds in a bespoke pair. It's worth it for the quality and finish and you'll find they last for years to come.

CROPPED TROUSERS

BEWARE! FLAPPY CROPPED TROUSERS ARE SO PROBLEMATIC. These are in my fashion sin bin but loads of women adore them. I just cannot understand their appeal. If you've got skinny legs, you look like you're coming out of a flower pot; if you're curvy, they hide the curves and make you look giant.

WIDE LEG

IDEALLY, YOU NEED TO BE TALL AND SLIM TO WEAR WIDE LEGS, otherwise they will create an blocky outline. 'Wide-leg, high-waisted trousers look great if you have a boyish figure and fairly long legs,' says Betty Jackson. 'But avoid this style if you are shorter than five foot four as it will make you look shorter still.

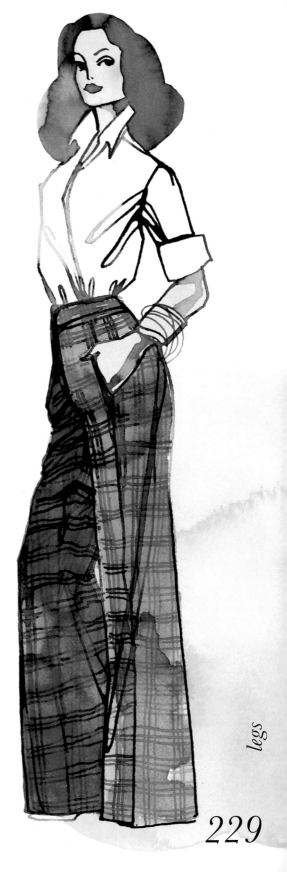

legs

229

Great _trousers_ to try . . .

1. Designer

- **NICOLE FARHI** – Great for top-quality trouser suits, slouchy wide-leg trousers and fine-tailored trousers in wool, tweed and cashmere.

- **MARGARET HOWELL** - Effortlessly stylish slouchy trousers that you can wear over and over again. Her Irish-linen trousers are great investment pieces.

- **DIANE VON FURSTENBERG** - Cuts for a woman's body and her GILLIGAN trousers fit beautifully on the leg and round the bottom, with a slight kick flare.

- **JOSEPH** - Designs beautifully cut trousers with a little stretch in them. Better for smaller frames as they tend to be cut very narrow.

- **SLACKS & CO** - Is an innovative new company that specializes in well-fitting women's trousers. The LAUREN trouser is a classic, slim, straight leg and has a bespoke quality and finish.

- **THEORY** - A US label that produces stylish trousers, good for office or casual wear. The ANAISS trousers are a gorgeous cut, and for designer trousers they're great value.

2. High street

- **FRENCH CONNECTION** - FCUK trousers are cut extremely well. Buy a size up sometimes so that they fit nicely on the hip. Both their slim-fit and wide-leg tailored trousers fit really well.

- **GAP** - Super value and flattering around the bottom and waist. Make sure you try them on and are happy with the fit.

- **M&S** - Their AUTOGRAPH classic wide-leg trousers fit snugly and are great value.

I seem to be on a permanent quest to find the perfect pair of trousers

- **<u>PRINCIPLES</u>** - Does a great long-leg black trouser, and flattering wide-leg jeans-style trousers.

- **<u>REISS</u>** - Nice-quality tailored trousers in wool gabardine and fine tweeds, fairly fashion-conscious but in great classic cuts.

- **<u>WALLIS</u>** - Excellent pinstripe straight-leg trousers, and slimming slant-pocket wide-leg jeans.

- **<u>ZARA</u>** - Makes great tailored trousers and also nice black, slim cigarette pants.

3. Investment office wear

- ARMANI EXCHANGE
- DIANE VON FURSTENBERG
- DKNY
- HUGO BOSS
- JAEGER
- JOSEPH
- NICOLE FARHI
- SLACKS & CO.
- SPORTMAX AND MAX MARA
- STELLA MCCARTNEY

4. High street buys

- AUTOGRAPH AT M&S
- DEBENHAMS
- FRENCH CONNECTION
- JIGSAW
- KAREN MILLEN
- NEXT
- MANGO
- REISS
- WAREHOUSE
- ZARA

legs

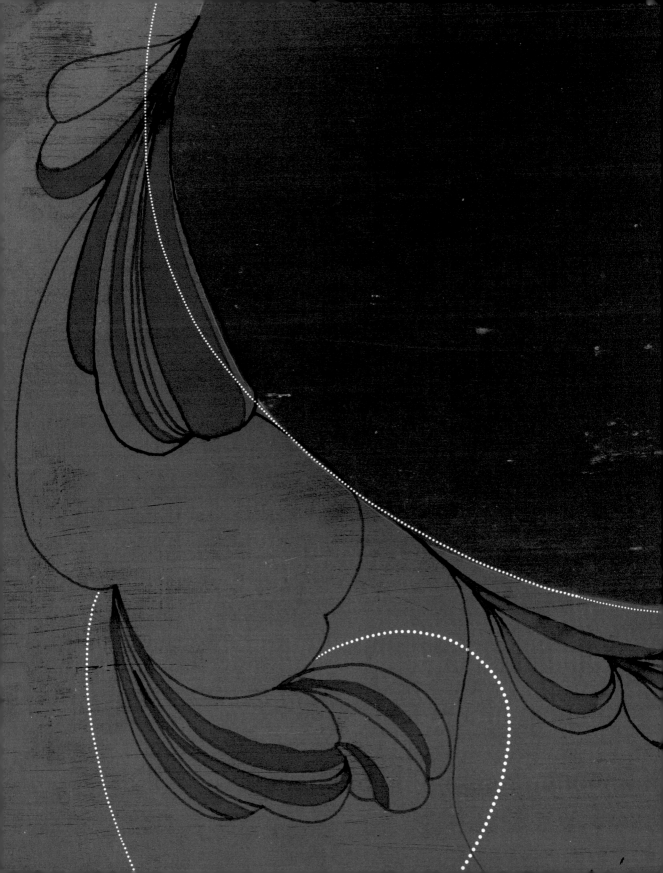

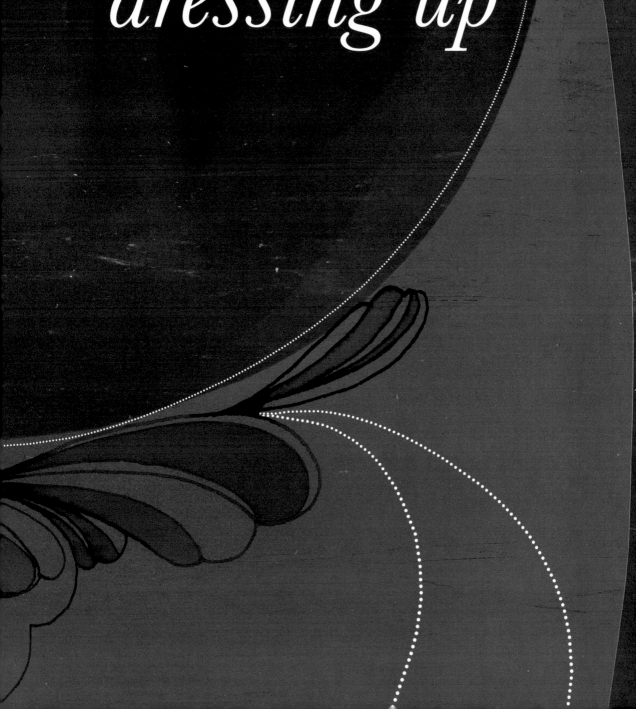

chapter nine
dressing up

evening wear

IN PRAISE OF THE TUXEDO

ONE OF MY BIG FAVOURITES FOR EVENING WEAR HAS ALWAYS BEEN A TUXEDO. IT ISN'T A LOOK EVERYONE CAN PULL OFF, MIND YOU. When I was still a teenager, Savile Row tailor-of-the-moment Tommy Nutter (and one of my best friends) made me the most incredible poppy-red, three-piece velvet tuxedo suit with grosgrain piping. I can't fit into it now, but have tucked it away in my wardrobe as it is the perfect example of menswear tailoring for women. One of the first men's suits I ever wore, it serves as a reminder that frocks are not always the best option when you're dressing for evening, especially for older women. Last year I found a similar jacket in Zara – what goes around comes around!

For me, a tuxedo is elegant, incredibly comfortable and a saving grace for us fortysome-things. God bless **YVES SAINT LAURENT** for designing the first tuxedo for women way back in the sixties. Certainly, if you're of the tallish, slenderish build, they are brilliant. If I have to go to a black-tie do, a tuxedo can be as beautiful as an evening dress. There are so many gorgeous ones, from **M&S** to **ZARA**, **YSL**, **EBAY** and – of course – charity shops. Very occasionally I'll dust off my white tailcoat, a costume made for me when I performed *My One and Only* on Broadway. Tailcoats are fun, but can be a bit theatrical.

I tend to wear tuxedo suits with a flat shoe, white shirt and – every now and then – a bow tie. Katharine Hepburn was the first to appropriate menswear all those years ago. It's a great look if you're not into frills, and I've never been a frilly girl. If you want to girlify a tuxedo suit, layer it beneath with a sequinned bustier or tunic top, a sparkly necklace or a chiffon blouse. If you're short, what the hell, wear a killer heel. It's a great way to give yourself height and a touch of class. Anyway, there's no such thing as sensible shoes. Flats can be just as sexy and perfect for evening as heels.

For me, the tuxedo is elegant, comfortable and a saving grace for us fortysomethings

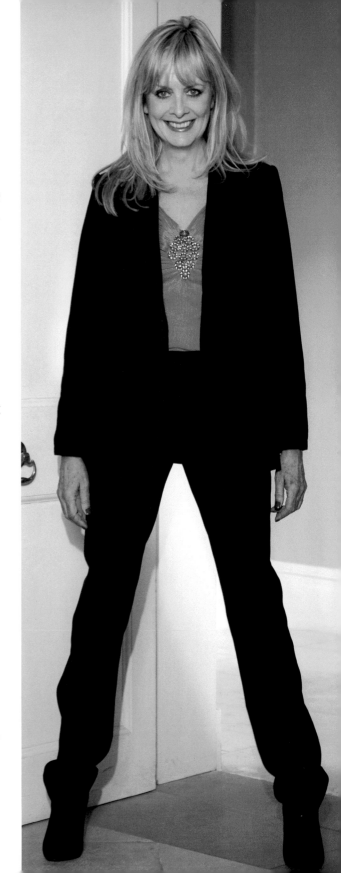

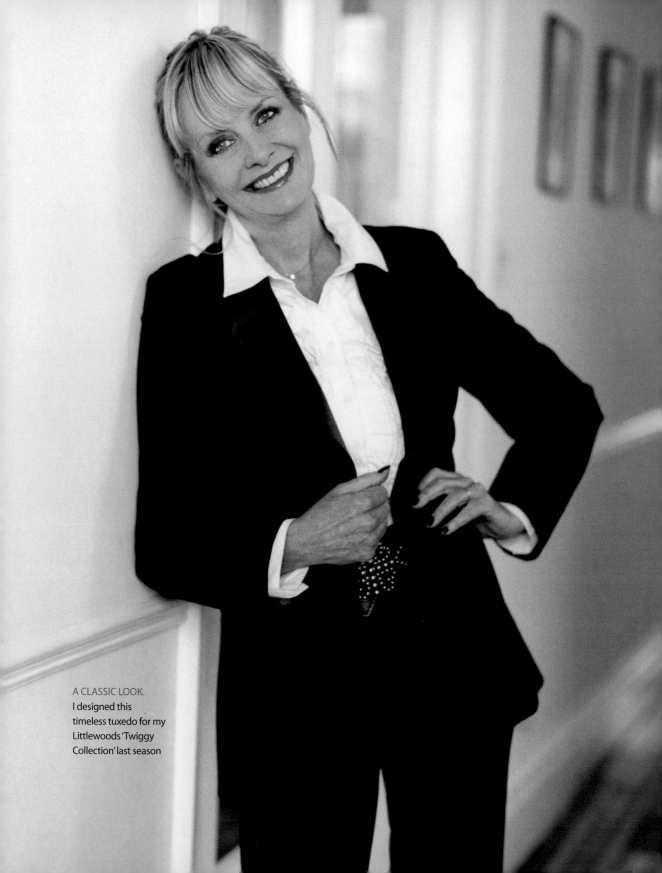

A CLASSIC LOOK.
I designed this
timeless tuxedo for my
Littlewoods 'Twiggy
Collection' last season

Great places to buy <u>tuxedos</u>

- **<u>JOSEPH</u>** – Usually has a great tuxedo suit with slim-line trousers and a satin stripe down the leg.

- **<u>JAEGER</u>** – Cuts a great velvet or wool tuxedo suit. Even buying a jacket and wearing it with your own jeans makes an innovative evening look.

- **<u>BY MALENE BIRGER</u>** – The **ELONGATED TUXEDO JACKET** with short lantern sleeves and single-button fastening looks classically stylish; wear with **PAUL & JOE** black silk wide-leg trousers.

- **<u>M&S</u>** – A good selection of tuxedos that look great for day and evening wear.

- **<u>GERARD DAREL</u>** – Cuts a mean smoking jacket and wide-leg trousers in black wool. It looks great worn with a dark sweater underneath.

- **<u>PRINCIPLES</u>** – Their black evening suit can be dressed up to look as good as a traditional tux.

- **<u>WALLIS</u>** – Known for well-fitting tuxedo jackets and matching trousers (look for these on the high street in the run-up to Christmas).

Or if you really want to push the boat out invest in a tailor-made suit from a man's tailor. Expensive – but you can't beat good tailoring.

dressing up

237

glam
it up

IF YOU ARE GOING TO A POSH DO AND WANT TO UP THE GLAMOUR STAKES, IT CAN STILL BE FUN TO WEAR A FROCK. What we really want in an evening dress is something made using beautiful fabric that that holds us in, enhances every curve and looks drop-dead gorgeous. It's always the women who are comfortable in what they are wearing who really stand out at a glam event. The women I always notice are elegantly dressed and aren't over the top. A true eccentric can get away with anything. But, for me, elegance is all about wearing beautiful fabrics, not flashing too much flesh, a little flourish of something sparkling.

The one thing you don't want is a cheap evening dress. It's tempting to go down that route, thinking you are only going to wear it once or twice a year. Sample sales can be a great place to find a knockout dress at a knock-down price. In an ideal world we're all after a couture gown! Couture dresses come with their own structured underwear to hoik you up, hold you in and stop everything from spilling out. Very few women can afford couture, but there's no harm in drawing inspiration from this rarefied end of the fashion world and applying it to your own budget. It all depends on the context of your night out.

dressing up

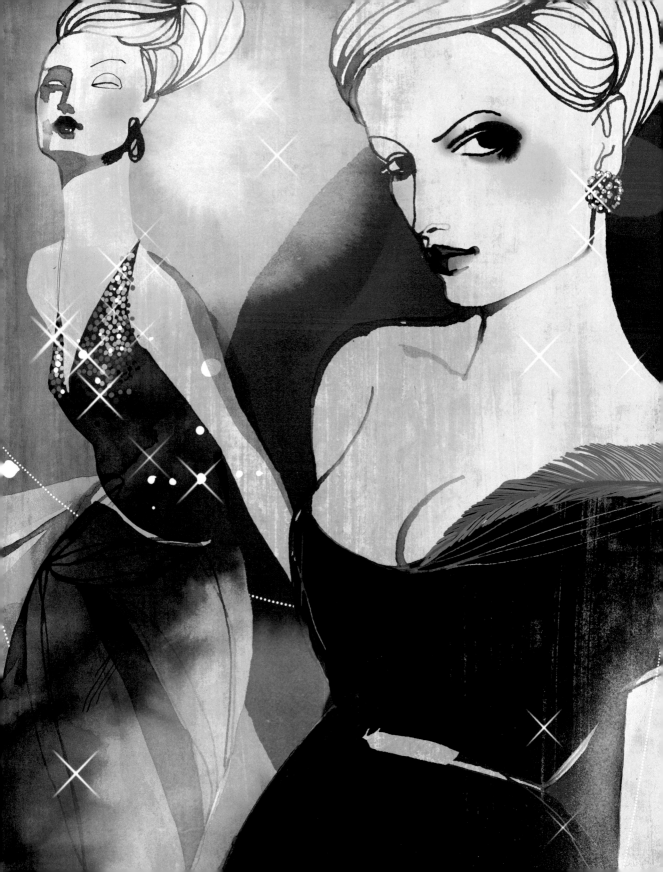

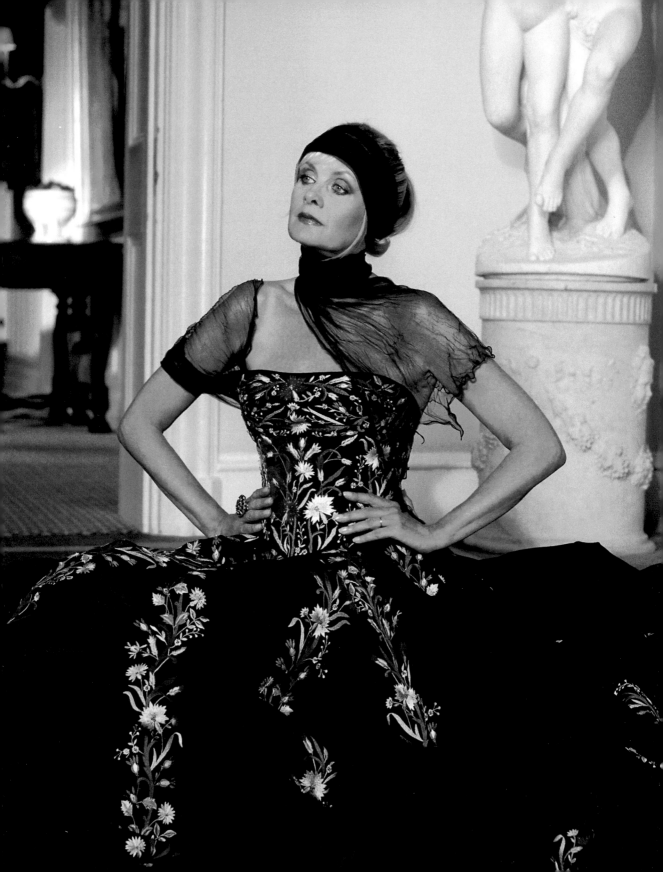

DRESSING TO GET NOTICED

IF YOU ARE HAVING A MILESTONE BIRTHDAY PARTY, OR YOU ARE GOING TO A POSH DO AND FANCY BEING THE CENTRE OF ATTENTION, PREPARE FOR A FULL-ON GETTING-READY EXTRAVAGANZA BEFORE YOU'VE EVEN LEFT THE FRONT DOOR. There's nothing like great hair and make-up to wow people and to help – whatever your outfit might be – add that little bit of extra polish. The trick with a great evening frock is to find something that cleverly distracts from any of the bits you don't like, and serves to seduce more by what it conceals than what it reveals.

And, anyway, who are we dressing for? Most women dress for other women. If you're single, then you might be thinking about dressing for men, or one particular lucky fella. There are many fortysomething women who find themselves on the singles circuit and haven't a clue what to wear on a hot date. After twenty-two years with my hubby I know what he likes and dislikes. So although I'm mostly dressing for me, I like to ask his opinion because I do enjoy dressing for him too.

One could spend a fortune on fashion and look so tacky and cheap. The truth is, no amount of money can ever buy you style. Fashion designer Betty Jackson knows a thing or two about dressing for evening. Her advice to us grown-up girls is: 'Don't be afraid!' Betty has lots of items from her own collection that would be suitable for any age. She has a word of advice before you embark on an evening-gown shopping spree. 'Look critically at both your back and front views in a long mirror and try to emphasize your good bits,' she suggests. 'Invest in shapes and silhouettes that suit both your shape and your lifestyle. Classic styles can always be updated with a fabulous new accessory.

Always go for quality not quantity and never forget: less is more

dressing up

241

Evening wear *dos* & *don'ts*

- **MAKE SURE** you've got enough time to get ready.

- **BOOK YOURSELF FOR A BLOW-DRY** if you have time, otherwise do it at home.

- **APPLY YOUR MAKE-UP** in good light.

- **PICK THE RIGHT FOOTWEAR.** If it's a sit-down dinner, towering heels will probably be fine, but they won't be if you're getting the bus home! If it's cocktails with lots of standing around, bear that in mind too. If your feet hurt, you'll be miserable all night.

- **AVOID CHILLY MOMENTS.** Pack a pashmina. You can always drape it over your shoulder or twist it around your evening-bag chain.

- **DON'T FORGET THE BENEFITS OF ADDING A FINISHING TOUCH** of a fab piece of jewellery. This can be costume or the real thing.

- **IF YOU PUT UP YOUR HAIR, CONSIDER THE BENEFITS OF A PAIR OF DROP EARRINGS.** This will elevate your look, especially if you have an off-the-shoulder dress.

- **DON'T OVERSTUFF YOUR EVENING BAG.** All you need is lipstick, tissues and some money, or at least your bus pass if you're lucky enough to have one!

Great <u>party frocks</u> to try . . .

1. Designer

- **<u>BROWNS</u>** – This London boutique has a dedicated evening-wear section and holds an impressive array of dresses by **BALENCIAGA**, **MISSONI** and **STELLA MCCARTNEY**.

- **<u>MATCHES</u>** – An innovative boutique with flagship stores in Wimbledon, Richmond and Notting Hill in London; their online boutique is equally dynamic, stocking fabulous evening wear by **BURBERRY PRORSUM**, **DIANE VON FURSTENBERG** and **LANVIN**.

- **<u>NET-A-PORTER</u>** – This internet-only boutique provides immaculate customer service and a wealth of designer dresses (look in the sale section for last-minute bargains).

- **<u>PRADA</u>** – If you're looking for an investment piece, a **PRADA** little black silk dress will be worth every penny.

- **<u>DIANE VON FURSTENBERG</u>** – Invest in a **DVF** jersey wrap dress and you won't look back.

- **<u>NICOLE FARHI</u>** – For classic evening shifts and bubble-hem dresses in silk or satin.

- **<u>JAEGER</u>** – Does a lovely collection of mid-length and full-length evening dresses.

2. High street

- **<u>COAST</u>** – For some of the best evening wear on the high street with matching accessories.

- **<u>DESIGNERS AT DEBENHAMS</u>** – Offers evening dresses from **BEN DE LISI**, **JASPER CONRAN** and **PEARCE FIONDA**. All are reasonably priced.

- **<u>MONSOON</u>** – Offers excellent embellished silk chiffon and satin evening dresses.

- **<u>M&S</u>** – I love M&S dresses. Their eveningwear, especially the Per Una limited edition range, can be exquisite.

OFF-THE-PEG OR MAKE YOUR OWN

Knitting is a great workout for your hands and it is so good for the brain

ANOTHER THING YOU COULD ALWAYS DO IS CREATE SOMETHING YOURSELF, IF, LIKE ME, YOU LOVE TO SEW. ONE OF MY GREAT PLEASURES IN LIFE IS TO GO FABRIC HUNTING. The best place in London for wonderful fabrics is Berwick Street. I can go there and rummage for hours and hours. When I have time, I love to sew. Recently, it's been curtains for the house, but if you've got a sewing machine and know your way around using patterns, you can make lovely things and save money at the same time. Also, you'll have a one-off creation.

For me, sewing is one of the most therapeutic ways to pass the time. My mum made all my clothes as a child and I have made lots for Carly over the years, including her graduation dress. I get my machine and fabric, crank up the music and it's the best. It's never too late to learn to sew. Knitting is also great and has become so fashionable as a hobby. In the 1970s I had a knitting machine and used to knit all my friends their Christmas presents. My friend Tracey Ullman is obsessed with knitting, and even published a book in 2006 on the subject, called *Knit 2 Together*. There are wonderful wool shops everywhere.

Needlepoint is lovely too. You can travel with it. There's nothing like making something to give yourself a boost. Until very recently, craft has been ignored. Currently, there's a huge craft renaissance, with knitting groups called Stitch 'n' Bitch, needlepoint workshops and sewing classes galore.

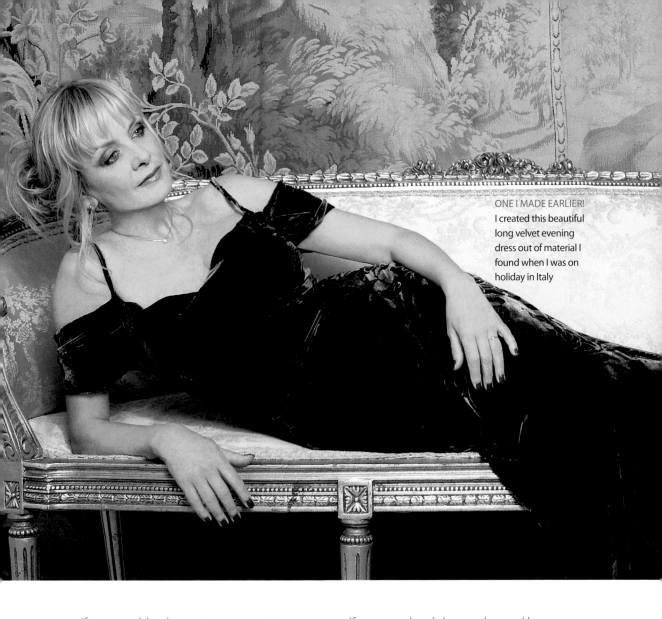

ONE I MADE EARLIER!
I created this beautiful
long velvet evening
dress out of material I
found when I was on
holiday in Italy

If you would rather not – or cannot – sew yourself, source a local dressmaker and have something made. A friend of mine was having a fiftieth birthday party recently and did just that, with huge success. For her, she said it was like choosing a wedding dress, but this time she could wear the outfit again and again. And why not? A bespoke frock may cost a few more pennies, but the fit of it will be perfect. To find a dressmaker near you, look in Yellow Pages or Google your area. Visit at least two, get a reference, check their portfolio and go for it. It's a sure guarantee you will look one hundred per cent original.

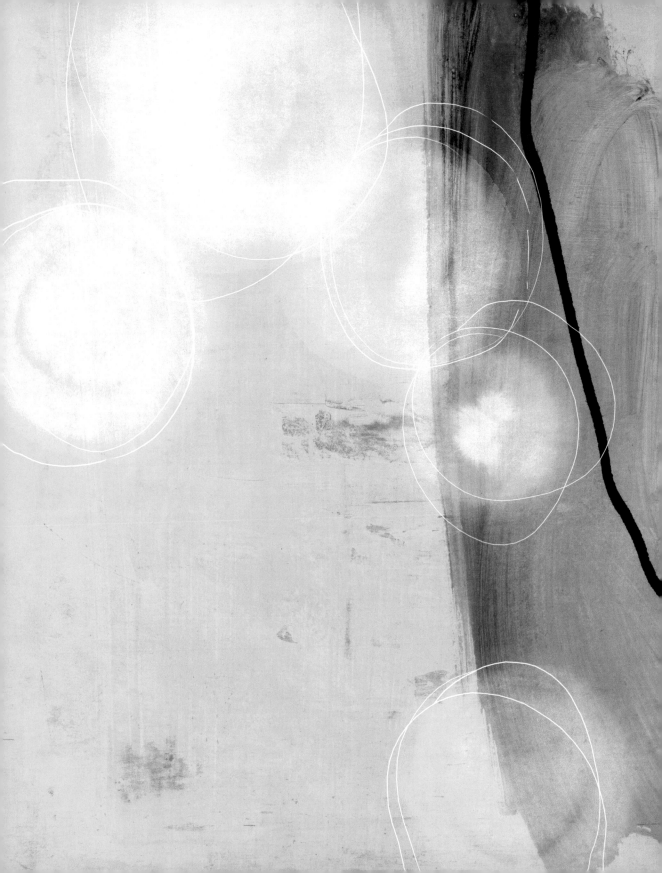

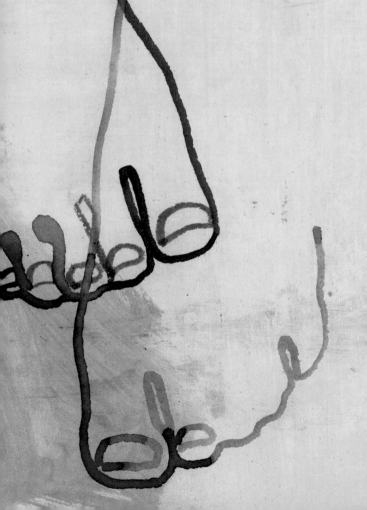

chapter ten
toes & feet

I INHERITED MY SMALL FEET FROM MY MUM. HERS WERE TINY. I DON'T MIND MY FEET, WHEREAS LOTS OF OTHER WOMEN I KNOW LOATHE THEIRS. From living in America for many years, where everyone has weekly pedicures, I got into the habit of having them once every month or so. Just make sure they are good salons, as non-trained pedicurists can be dangerous.

We spend our lives on our feet, and by the time we reach our forties plus, it can often take a lot of soul-searching (ha ha) to feel okay about baring them in the summer months. If you can, do have regular pedicures. Regular appointments with an expert will help to keep your feet in check, spot ingrowing toenails and other hazards. Poor circulation can become an issue as we get older, which is why a good old scrub with a body brush on the soles of the feet can be an excellent addition to your daily shower. I love treating my feet after a shower to a good slathering of foot cream. It's also amazing what a weekly exfoliation with a loofah or pumice stone, followed by DIY foot massage at home, can do for those dry heels and ankles. I also try not to wear the same pair of shoes two days running. If you alternate your shoes, they will last longer and – in summer months, when feet sweat much more – this helps to keep shoes from becoming damp and niffy.

toes & feet

For overall health and well-being, it is so important to look after your feet

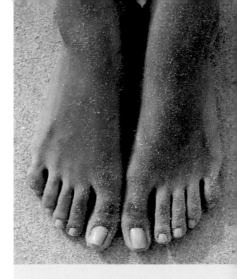

One of the best things in the world is to feel the sand between your toes. Walking barefoot is one of life's simple pleasures. I adore it. It's the best natural exfoliant too! Another treat is reflexology. This is a complementary therapy that works on the feet or hands. It eases tension, boosts circulation and is said to be a way in which blockages can be released to restore the free flow of energy to the whole body. To find a reflexologist near you, go to the **ASSOCIATION OF REFLEXOLOGISTS** at **www.aor.org.uk**.

I love having bright nail polish on my toes for summer. Salon pedicures are a fab treat, but you can just as easily pamper your feet at home. Having said that, it can be tricky to paint your toenails. I know I find it hard. The most boring thing is waiting for polish to dry. Use toe dividers or cotton-wool balls between the toes.

FOOT TREATS
YOU MIGHT
LIKE TO TRY

LUXURY
- *Margaret Dabbs Intensive Treatment Foot Oil*

MIDDLE
- *DDF Pedi-Cream*
- *Origins Reinventing the Heel™ Mega-Moisture*

BUDGET
- *Sally Hansen Pedicure in a Minute*
- *Weleda Foot Balm*

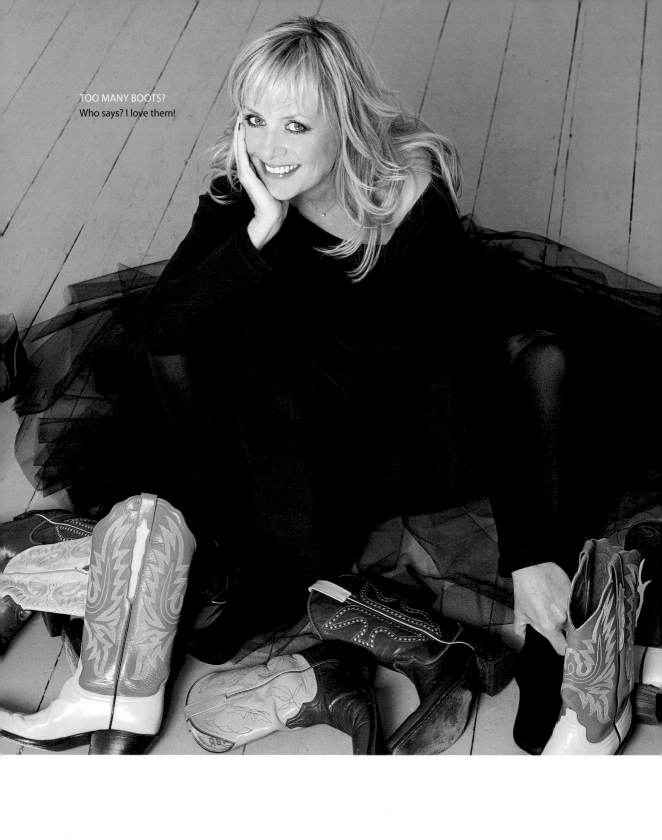

TOO MANY BOOTS?
Who says? I love them!

boots

I'VE ALREADY CONFESSED THAT I'M A BOOTAHOLIC. I'M NOT TELLING YOU HOW MANY PAIRS I HAVE AS I HAVE LOST COUNT. One of my favourites is a pair of soft-leather swashbucklers, bought in the 1980s. My daughter Carly has one of my other fave pairs in moss-green suede. For years and years I lived in another pair, up to the knee, with diamanté studs around the top and a tie at the back, in soft black suede. In the nineties they just weren't fashionable, so one day I decided to chuck them out and took them to the local charity shop. Let's hope somebody else is having a lovely time wearing those boots as, if not, I'll wrestle them back! I have missed them ever since.

Boots can look great teamed with full skirts, or skinny jeans tucked in, if you're confident enough to wear skinnies, that is. They also look fab with boot-cut trousers.

COWBOY BOOTS

I DON'T CARE IF THEY'RE NOT TRENDY, I LOVE COWBOY BOOTS. I BOUGHT MY FIRST PAIR IN 1972 IN LOS ANGELES. They were tan and brown, very traditional, as back then that's all you could get. I've worn them with jeans and long gypsy skirts. In fact my daughter still wears them now. Anyone can wear them, not just tall people. They bring enough height to make you swing those hips a bit without running the risk of falling flat on your face owing to them being too dainty. And they are incredibly comfortable – I can walk for miles in mine.

toes & feet

251

When I see a pair of boots I love, it's very hard for me to walk away

<u>GOOD FOR</u> Full skirts and jeans.

<u>TO BUY</u>
1. **R.SOLES** – The best range of authentic North American hand-tooled leather cowboy boots – an institution in itself.

2. **OFFICE** – A classic cowboy boot is usually available in their autumn/winter collections.

3. **VINTAGE COWBOY BOOTS** can be found in charity shops and specialist vintage shops.

KNEE-HIGH CHUNKY-HEELED BOOTS

<u>GOOD FOR</u> Jersey dresses and tights, winter dresses if worn with woolly tights, and for tucking jeans into.

<u>TO BUY</u>
1. **NEXT** – Offer good-looking, chunky wooden-heel, pull-on boots in black or chocolate leather.

2. **M&S** – Super-value, knee-high boots.

3. **PIED À TERRE** – Stylish and functional; look for attractive details like side-stitching and buckles.

4. **RUSSELL & BROMLEY** – Classic, good-quality boots. They are not cheap but if you buy a traditional style or colour, like a rich tan or black patent, they'll continue to look great winter after winter.

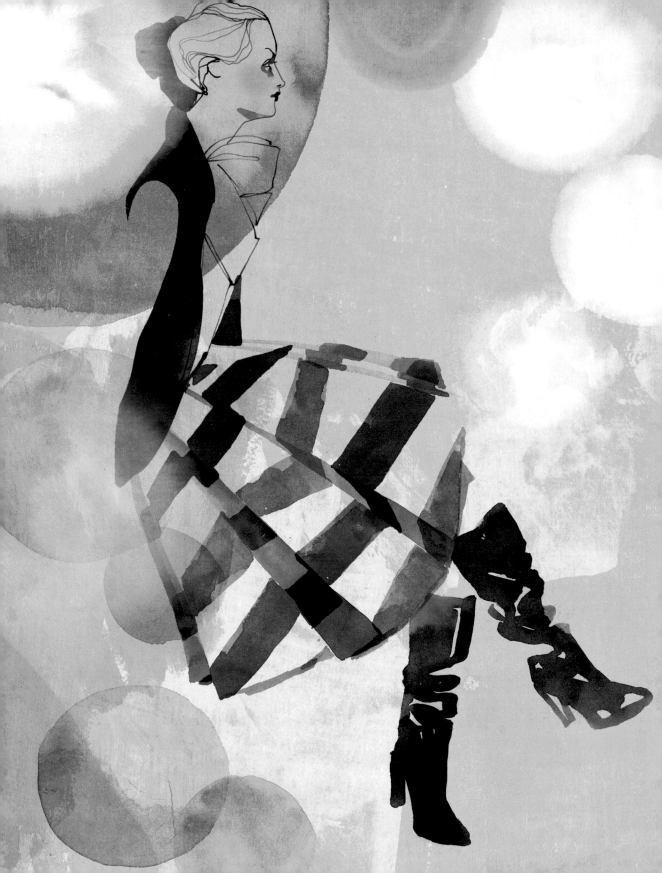

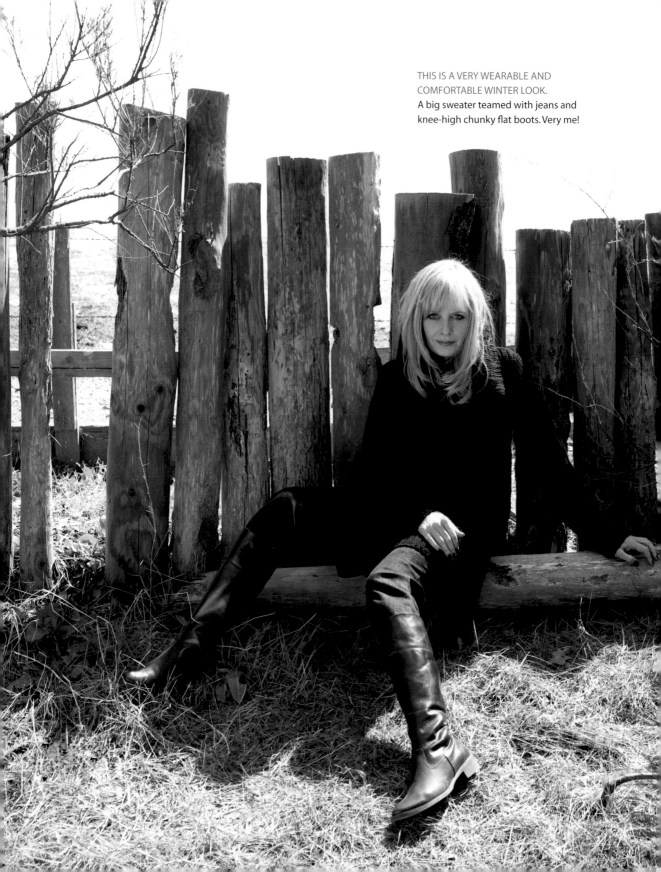

THIS IS A VERY WEARABLE AND
COMFORTABLE WINTER LOOK.
A big sweater teamed with jeans and
knee-high chunky flat boots. Very me!

KNEE-HIGH FLAT BOOTS

<u>GOOD FOR</u> Skirts in winter, slim-fit jeans/cords worn tucked in.

<u>TO BUY</u>
1. ANGELINE TOURNIER – A specialist shoe designer who makes shoes and boots with an extra-wide fitting. The bonus is that despite the width they still look fashionable and stylish, which isn't often the case with wider-fit footwear. The black riding boot is a winner.

2. ARCHE – Super-comfortable flat, suede, rubber-soled boots. You can walk all day in them without discomfort.

3. HOBBS – A classic British brand. Their flat winter boots are well-made and sturdy.

4. RUSSELL & BROMLEY – They do a great flat pull-on boot that is comfortable and stylish.

SHOE BOOTS & ANKLE BOOTS

<u>SHOE BOOTS ARE GOOD FOR</u> jeans and smart black/dark trousers.

<u>ANKLE BOOTS ARE GOOD FOR</u> slim-limbed or younger women. These are tricky because they can be foreshortening on the leg. Best left to the young unless you go for slouchy, suede/soft boots.

<u>TO BUY</u>
1. ALDO – This Spanish high-street shop offers fashion-led shoe boots at reasonable prices.

2. OFFICE – For great little cut-off ankle boots.

3. DUNE – For kitten-heel shoe boots in patent or leather.

toes & feet

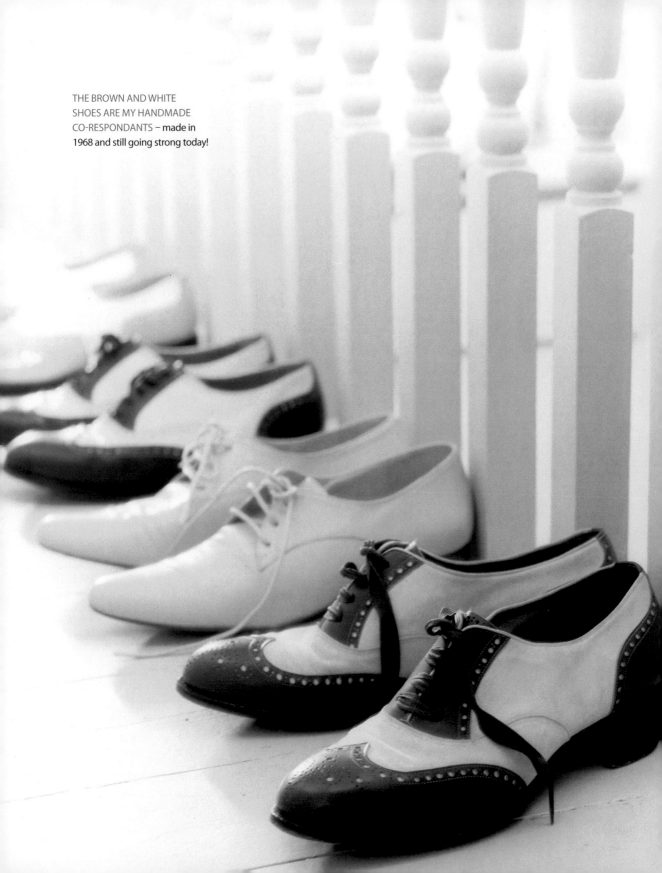

THE BROWN AND WHITE
SHOES ARE MY HANDMADE
CO-RESPONDANTS – made in
1968 and still going strong today!

shoes

FLAT SHOES

I LOVE FLAT SHOES, MORE SO THAN HEELS, EVEN THOUGH I HAVE TONS OF HEELS CLUTTERING UP MY WARDROBE. One of my obsessions is men's correspondent lace-ups. They're very now, but I have worn them for years. They are incredibly comfortable. Back in the sixties I had a couple of pairs made at a gentlemen's shoemakers in Cork Street, the only place to find them. I was the shop's first female customer! They are still in my wardrobe today. I love them. **ROBERT CLERGERIE**, **SISLEY**, **CHURCHES** and **HOBBS** are great places to seek them out. I call them my Fred Astaire shoes. I could walk forever in them, and always travel with at least one pair.

Women and shoes go together like tea and biscuits. We shall always love them and they shall always bring us joy

toes & feet

257

There are no rules about shoes in my book. They are one of the few things we can all wear and enjoy

I also love ballet pumps. They are the dream shoes because they are so comfortable. They came back in fashion a few years ago and thankfully are still widely available on the high street. Ballet pumps look great with jeans and summer dresses; you can even wear the right pair with an evening dress.

You won't often find me in a pair of killer heels. My heel height doesn't rise above two and a half inches as I would just fall over! I have friends who can wear heels much higher, though. Depending on your pain threshold, you may be able to wear heels from dawn till dusk. I can't be dealing with agonizing feet, but will make an exception if I'm going to a swanky party.

Great _flat shoes_ to try . . .

1. Ballet flats

- **ARCHE** – This French footwear company designs the most comfortable footwear. The Arche Sagone is a round-toed, ballerina-style flat shoe with excellent support and cushioning (this is often missing in regular ballet flats).

- **FRENCH SOLE** – The traditional home of the ballerina flat. They are now available in an enormous range of colours, textures and fits, and are perfect for everyday wear with trousers, jeans and skirts.

- **LANVIN** – For a designer fix, these luxury, flat, banana-shaped pumps are divine.

- **LA REDOUTE** – This mail-order catalogue offers a good range of ballerinas and flat pumps that are accessible and affordable.

- **PRETTY BALLERINAS** – A great website for top-quality ballet flats. Available in patent, suede, leather and cotton in a huge range of colours and patterns.

- **RUSSELL & BROMLEY** – Ballet flats in classic patent, coloured leather, metallic gold and silver.

- **TOD'S** – The makers of the driving shoe do a super range of flat lace-ups, banana- shaped ballerina flats and loafers too.

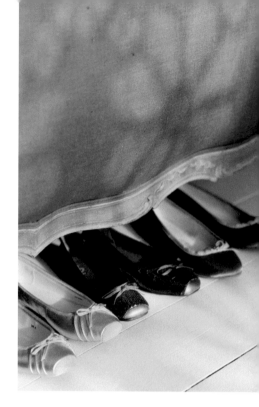

2. Moccasins (an ultra comfy alternative to the ballet flat), brogues & flat lace-ups

- **WWW.MINNETONKA.CO.UK** – Offers a great range of classic leather and suede moccasins, loafers and fringed boots.

- **CAR SHOE** – Luxurious yet practical shoes from the makers of Prada. Their classic lace-ups are fabulous.

- **FRATELLI ROSSETTI** – Superb quality, Italian, leather lace-up shoes including loafers, courts and brogues.

- **RUSSELL & BROMLEY** – Usually have a traditional lace-up or brogue-style winter shoe.

- **HOBBS** – For well-made classic English lace-ups that are perfect with trousers.

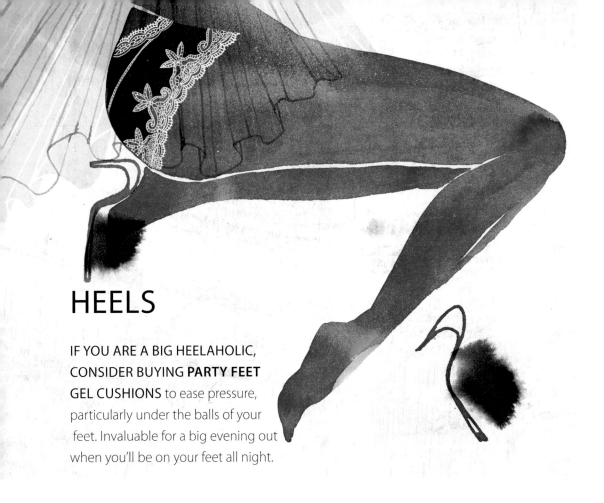

HEELS

IF YOU ARE A BIG HEELAHOLIC, CONSIDER BUYING **PARTY FEET GEL CUSHIONS** to ease pressure, particularly under the balls of your feet. Invaluable for a big evening out when you'll be on your feet all night.

Great __heels__ to try . . .

- **<u>CHRISTIAN LOUBOUTIN</u>** – Their distinctive red soles will certainly get you noticed. Chic styles, shapes and colours available. The classic patent, round-toe courts are amazing and a worthy investment.

- **<u>DUNE</u>** – Their signature pointed-toe heels offer great value for money.

- **<u>JIMMY CHOO</u>** – Super-stylish and sexy, these heels have their own distinctive style. The pointed-toe courts and high strappy sandals are superb.

- **<u>L. K. BENNETT</u>** – Always has a fabulous range of evening heels in satin with bows and diamanté clasps, which are great for special occasions.

- **MANOLO BLAHNIK** – The crème de la crème of heels, they are well balanced and in butter-soft kid leather and suede. One **MANOLO** purchase will last a lifetime.

- **PRADA** – You can usually find something classic but stylish, whether you're looking for an evening sandal or a daytime court shoe.

SLIPPERS

Great <u>slippers</u> to try . . .

- **CELTIC SHEEPSKIN** – The British alternative to **UGG AUSTRALIA**. Their **LOUNGER MOCCASIN** is an extremely plush and fluffy traditional slipper, and the **CELT MULE** is a simple slip-on. Competitively priced, and come in an array of colours.

- **HOLISTIC SILK** – The angora and wool **SLIPPER SOCKS** come complete with a padded sole, perfect for walking around the house, while the **HOLISTIC SILK BROCADE MASSAGING** and **MAGNETIC SLIPPERS** have a specially fitted insole that gives you a lovely reflexology foot massage.

- **THE WHITE COMPANY** – Fully washable, classic white-cotton waffle slippers.

SHEEPSKIN BOOTS

Great <u>sheepskin boots</u> to try . . .

- **LOVE FROM AUSTRALIA** – Similar to **UGGS** but have a larger range of other styles including Nappa leather sheepskin-lined boots.

- **UGG BOOTS** – The **CLASSIC SHORT** boots in chocolate or black, are super-cosy.

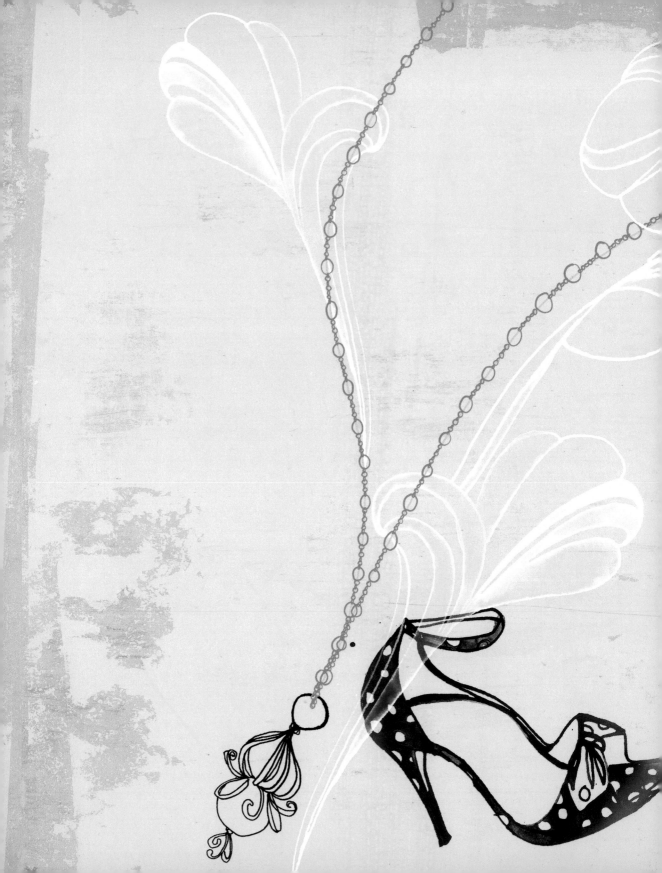

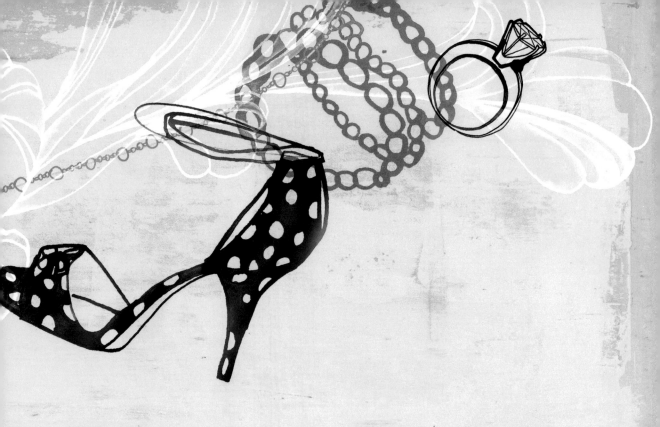

chapter eleven
accessories

handbags

IN THE SIXTIES, MOST WOMEN OWNED JUST ONE OR TWO HANDBAGS. NOT SO THESE DAYS. In the last few years, handbag one-upmanship has become a professional sport among women. The ultimate style trophy, a great handbag can be a way for women to reference high fashion without slavishly dressing from head to toe in the latest trends. If you're a bit shy about changing your way of dressing, and prefer instead to stick to what you know, buying a mad handbag is a fab way to update your entire wardrobe. Choose carefully. If you're going to spend your hard-earned money on a great bag, test how heavy it is. So many 'it' bags weigh a ton – they can wreak havoc on your neck and shoulder muscles. I love bags with practical touches. I have a couple of the ridiculously priced designer bags. If you want to spend that money, it's up to you. I love my handbags, not quite as much as I love my boots and shoes, but almost.

I must confess to owning quite a few bags and love to wear them as part of an outfit

accessories

264

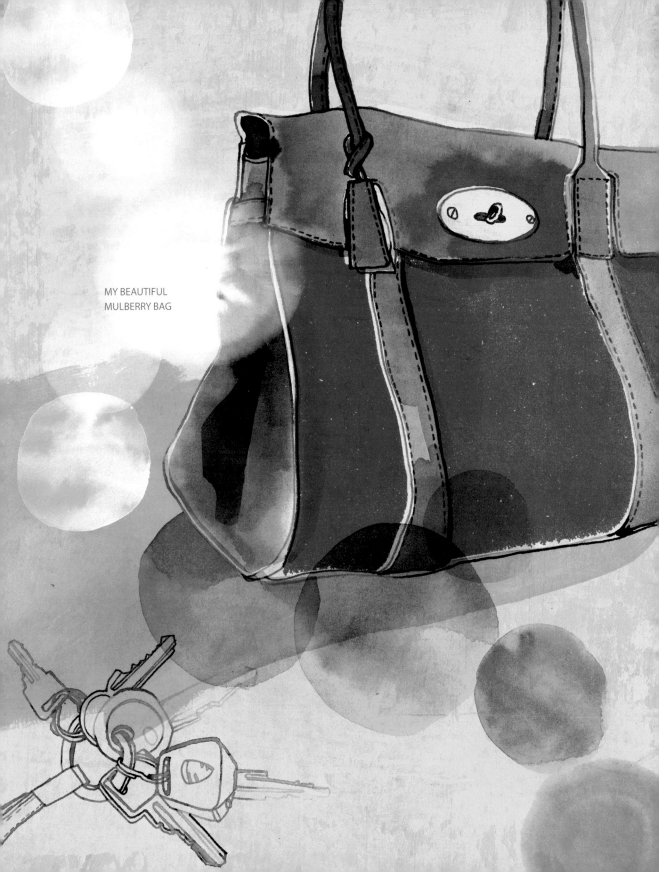

MY BEAUTIFUL
MULBERRY BAG

If you don't have the cash to splash, you don't have to go down the designer route to find a great bag. Carly has bought beautiful leather bags from charity shops. It is always worth spending a few quid on something that has good quality. You don't need lots of money to be stylish. You really don't. Charity shops and antique fairs are also where you'll find a good evening bag. I have a small collection of beaded ones from the 1920s. You can also buy amazing ones from shops like **ACCESSORIZE**.

Great <u>labels</u> for gorgeous bags

- <u>**ANYA HINDMARCH**</u> – Her shopping totes are understated yet gorgeous, in a ddition to a variety of stylish over-the-shoulder bags in leather and patent, and a wealth of satin evening clutches.

- <u>**BILL AMBERG**</u> – Makes butter-soft leather satchels and suede slouchy bags that are definitely an indulgent investment.

- <u>**CHANEL**</u> – The classic quilted, gilt-chain-strap bag will always be the height of chic!

- <u>**JOHN LEWIS**</u> – Try their school department: there's nothing like a satchel for an understated classic leather bag.

- <u>**LITTLEWOODS DIRECT**</u> – I designed the **TWIGGY LEATHER TOTE** for **LITTLEWOODS DIRECT**. It's a gorgeous toffee-brown leather shopper, and, as with all simple leather bags, it will age well. There is also the **TWIGGY LARGE LEATHER TASSLE BAG**.

- <u>**MULBERRY**</u> – Their **BAYSWATER** is a fabulous shape, and the oak leather lasts forever.

- <u>**ORLA KIELY**</u> – This Irish designer has cornered the market in bags. They can be found in interesting clothes boutiques nationwide. They are quirky yet long lasting, available in rich olive, chocolate and black leather, or brightly coloured laminated canvas prints.

- <u>**RADLEY**</u> – For coloured-leather totes, workbags, wallets and purses, this British leather-goods company has plenty to offer.

hats

I LOVE HATS AND WEAR THEM ALL THE TIME IN WINTER. MY MUM ALWAYS SAID, 'IF YOU KEEP YOUR HEAD WARM, IT KEEPS YOU WARM.' I love knitted skullcaps, beanies, cloche hats, trilbys, soft-felt fedoras. Berets are fab and I wear them often. There's no age limit on hats. In summer it's mainly baseball caps, especially for holidays, to keep the sun out of my eyes. If it's roasting hot, then there's nothing like a battered old straw sunhat to stave off the strong rays. It's ironic that the sixties killed the hat for women and for men. Before the decade that changed the world, if a woman was going out, she wasn't dressed unless she had on a hat and gloves. It does get harder as you get older to wear a hat without looking too costumey, but why not! Or you can buy wonderful feathers to clip into the hair. Sometimes, I create a 1920s look by pinning a ribbon round the crown of my head. It's lovely for a posh evening out.

www.hatsandthat.com is a useful website for all things hat-related.

Hats are really rather wonderful. I love it when I see somebody all dressed up with a hat

accessories

267

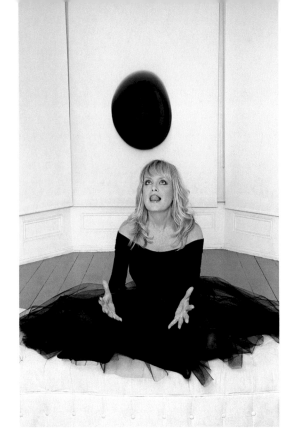

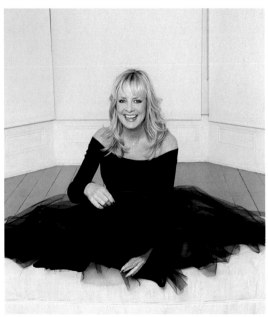

Great <u>hats</u> to try . . .

1.   Berets

- KANGOL

2.   Wool hats

- BRORA
- JIGSAW
- JO GORDON
- LAND'S END

3.   Formal hats

- ACCESSORIZE
- COZMO JENKS
- DESIGNERS AT DEBENHAMS
- JAEGER
- JAMES LOCK & CO
- HOUSE OF FLORA
- LIBERTY
- PHASE EIGHT
- STEPHEN JONES

4.   Trilby hats

- ACCESSORIZE
- ASOS
- FRED BARE
- FRENCH CONNECTION
- TED BAKER

I bought this black bowler hat to wear with a man's suit and ended up wearing it with this evening skirt

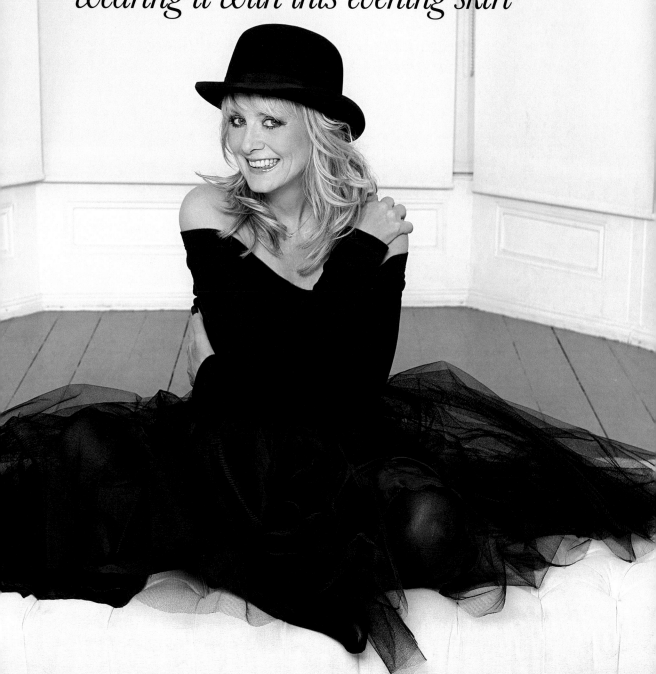

jewels

IF YOU'VE GOT ANY ROCKS – COSTUME JEWELLERY OR REAL DIAMONDS – NOW IS THE TIME TO SHOW THEM OFF. I love antique jewellery, especially art nouveau, art deco, Victorian and Georgian period. These styles I much prefer to modern-looking jewellery. I love choker necklaces. Sitting on the neckline, they can look very sexy. Pearls with a little black dress is an unbeatable combination, as proven by Audrey Hepburn. What I love is that the world is your oyster with jewellery, whether you're lucky enough to have the real thing, or you like to have fun on the high street. I've got plastic beads and bracelets which I adore as much as more grown-up, ladylike pieces.

Obviously, don't wear your best diamonds out shopping, but for a special night out, a diamond can add that much-needed polish. The same applies to a chunky gold bracelet. Boot fairs and antique fairs are great places to find costume jewellery. My sister-in-law bought what she was told was a fake gold necklace for a few pounds at a boot fair recently, and lucked out. It turned out to be worth a few hundred. The most important thing, regardless of price, is to buy what you like. My mum always wore a brooch and loved marquesite, which is very pretty and often found at antique fairs, and not too expensive either.

A paste brooch or something diamanté can be a lovely way to dress up a simple shirt or jacket

Great <u>jewellery</u> to try . . .

1. Costume jewellery

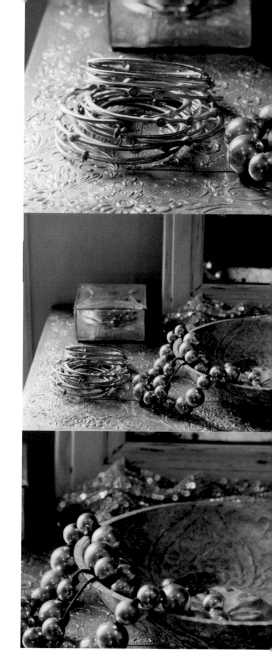

- <u>**JIGSAW**</u> – has lovely one-off pieces: chains, rings, pendants that are very flattering

- <u>**JAEGER**</u> – does stylish costume jewellery, not too expensive

- <u>**CHANEL**</u> – costume jewellery – very expensive

- <u>**ADELE MARIE**</u> – is fab for chunky rings and bangles

- <u>**WWW.TREASUREBOX.CO.UK**</u> – a great website for reasonable costume jewellery

2. Splurge jewellery

- LINKS OF LONDON – for great gold and silver charm bracelets
- COLEMAN DOUGLAS PEARLS – for pearls
- TIFFANY & CO – for silver
- DINNY HALL – for silver
- GEORG JENSEN – for silver
- SOLANGE AZAGURY-PARTRIDGE – for incredible statement pieces and bespoke service
- S J PHILLIPS – for the most beautiful collection of antique jewellery in the UK

accessories

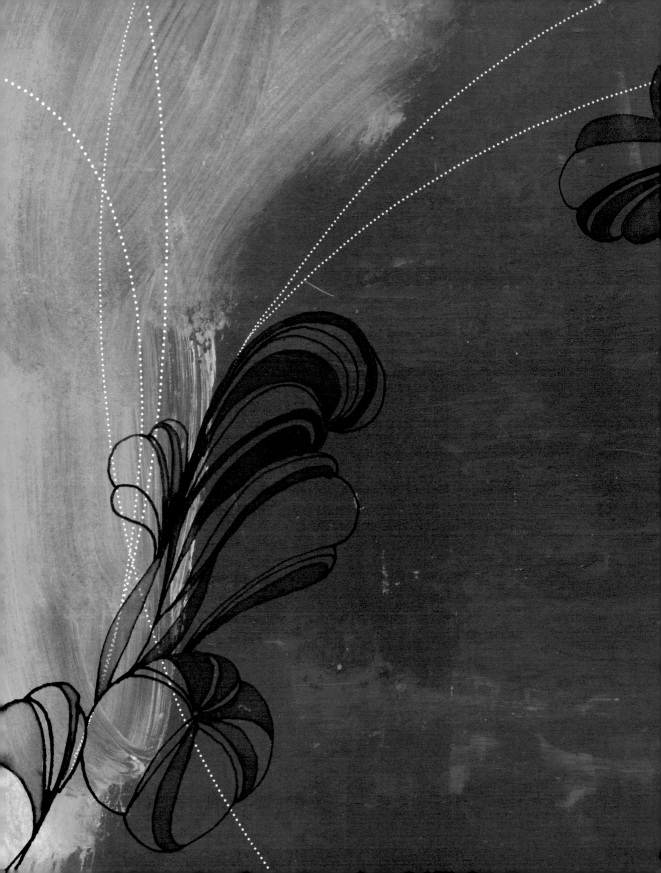

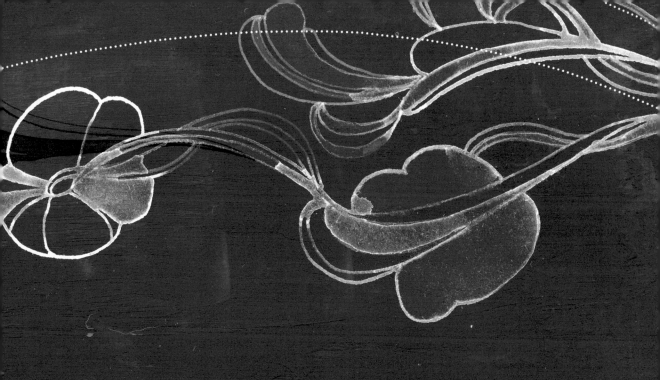

conclusion

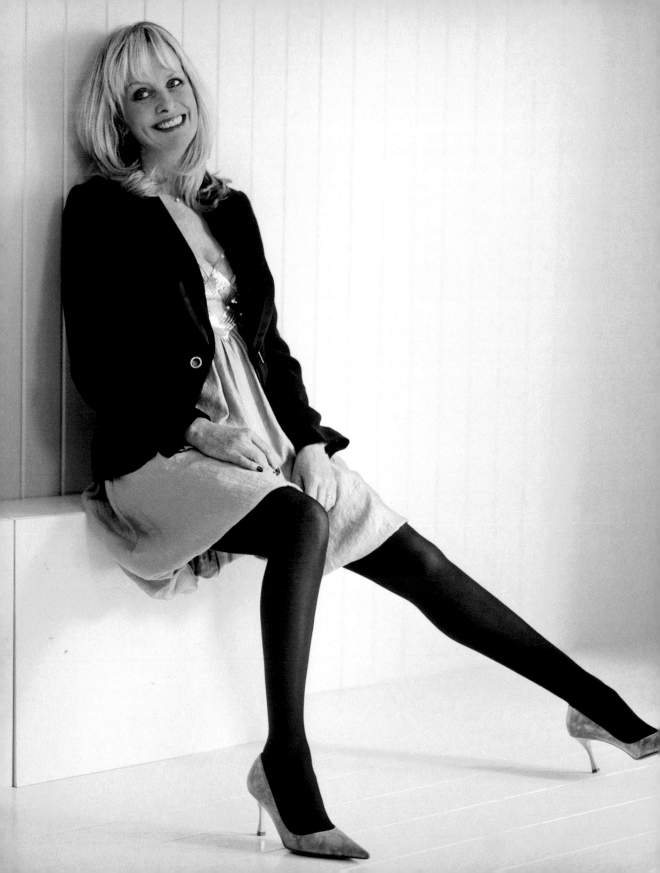

W

WELL, I HOPE YOU HAVE ENJOYED READING THIS BOOK, AND THAT IT HAS GIVEN YOU FOOD FOR THOUGHT AND ENCOURAGED YOU TO TRY NEW THINGS. REMEMBER, FASHION SHOULD BE FUN.

Go and have that new hair cut or colour or both! Cheer yourself up with trying new things, new looks; there's something out there for everyone.

Join an exercise class or dance class. I promise you, you will benefit from the results. And most importantly, have a good look at your diet – remember, you are what you eat!

So don't think about it – start right NOW!

Thanks for reading.

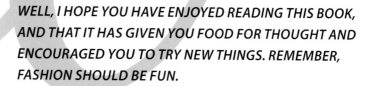

where to buy

FASHION

_A_CCESSORIZE 0870 412 9000
www.accessorize.co.uk
ADELE MARIE 020 8440 1687
www.adelemarie.com
AGNÈS B 020 7935 5556
www.agnesb.com
ALBERTA FERRETTI 020 7235 2349
ALDO 020 7836 7692
 www.aldoshoes.com
ALL SAINTS 0870 412 9000
ALLEGRA HICKS 020 7235 8989
www.allegrahicks.com
AMERICAN APPAREL 020 7734 4477
www.americanapparel.com
ANGELINE TOURNIER
www.angelinetournier.com
ANYA HINDMARCH 020 7838 9177
www.anyahindmarch.com
A.P.C. 020 7221 7070 www.apc.fr
ARCHE www.thenaturalshoestore.com
ARISTOC 01623 444 299
www.tightsplease.co.uk

www.mytights.com
ARMANI EXCHANGE 020 7479 7760
ARMANI JEANS 020 7491 8080
ASICS www.milletsports.co.uk
ASOS www.asos.com

_B_ENETTON 0845 389 9455
BENTALLS 020 8456 1001
www.bentalls.co.uk
BETTY JACKSON 020 7589 7884
www.my-wardrobe.com
BHS 0845 196 0000
BILL AMBERG 020 7727 3560
www.billamberg.com
BODAS 020 7229 4464
www.bodas.co.uk
BODEN 0845 677 5000
www.boden.co.uk
BRAZA www.brazabra.com
BRIONI 020 7491 7700
BRORA 020 7736 9944
www.brora.co.uk

BURBERRY 07000 785676
BY MALENE BIRGER
www.my-wardrobe.com

_C_+C CALIFORNIA Harvey Nichols
020 7235 5000; Selfridges 0800 123 400
CALVIN KLEIN UNDERWEAR
020 7290 5900; www.figleaves.com
CAMPER 020 7409 3130
www.camper.com
CAR SHOE CONNOLLY
020 7439 2510
CARVELA 0845 257 2571
www.kurtgeiger.com
CELINE 020 7297 4999
CELTIC SHEEPSKIN CO 01637 871605
www.celtic-sheepskin.co.uk
CHANEL 020 7493 5040
www.chanel.com
CHARLES & PATRICIA LESTER
01873 855115
www.charles-patricia-lester.co.uk

CHARLES TYRWHITT 0845 337 4337
www.ctshirts.co.uk
CHARNOS www.tightsplease.co.uk
CHRISTIAN LOUBOUTIN
020 7245 6510
CHURCH'S 020 7734 2438
www.church-footwear.com
COAST 01865 881986
www.coast-stores.co.uk
COLEMAN DOUGLAS PEARLS
020 7373 3369
www.passion4pearls.com
COMMANDO Debenhams stores
nationwide & www.figleaves.com
COMPTOIR DES COTONNIERS
www.comptoirdescotonniers.com
COZMO JENKS 020 7258 0111
www.cozmojenks.co.uk

*D*EBENHAMS 08445 616161
www.debenhams.com
DIANE VON FURSTENBERG
0800 121 8949 www.dvflondon.com
DINNY HALL 020 7588 9192
www.dinnyhall.co.uk
DKNY 020 7499 6238 www.dkny.com
DOLCE & GABBANA 020 7659 9000
DONNA KARAN 020 7479 7900
DOROTHY PERKINS 0845 121 4515
www.dorothyperkins.co.uk
DUNE 020 7258 3605 www.dune.co.uk

*E*GG 36 Kinnerton Street, London
SW1 020 7235 9315
ELIXIR www.rigbyandpeller.com
ELLE MACPHERSON INTIMATES
Debenhams stores nationwide &
www.figleaves.com
ESPRIT 020 7025 7700
EVANS 0845 121 4516 www.evans.co.uk

F&F COLLECTION (Tesco Clothing)
0800 505 555

FALKE 020 7493 8442
www.mytights.com
FANTASIE www.figleaves.com
FASHION FIRST AID
www.figleaves.com
FASHION FORMS www.figleaves.
FAYREFORM www.figleaves.com
FENN WRIGHT & MANSON
020 8948 4158
www.fennwrightmanson.com
FENWICK 020 629 9161
FRATELLI ROSETTI 020 7259 6397
FRED BARE 01904 624 579
FREDA (MATCHES) 020 7221 0255
www.matchesfashion.com
FREEMANS 0800 900 200
www.freemans.com
FRENCH CONNECTION
020 7036 7200 www.fcukbymail.com
FRENCH SOLE 01189 888800
www.frenchsole.com
FREYA 01536 764 334
www.figleaves.com

*G*AP 0800 427 789 www.gap.com
GEORG JENSEN 020 7499 6541
GEORGE AT ASDA 0500 100 055
GEORGINA VON ETZDORF
www.gve.co.uk
GERARD DAREL FENWICK
020 7629 9161
GIORGIO ARMANI 020 235 6232
GOTTEX www.figleaves.com

H&M 020 7323 2211
HANRO Harrods 020 7730 1234
www.figleaves.com
HARRODS 020 7730 1234
HARVEY NICHOLS 020 7235 5000
HATS AND THAT www.hatsandthat.com
HEIDI KLEIN 0845 206 2000
www.heidiklein.co.uk
HI-TEC www.milletsports.co.uk

HOBBS 020 7586 5550
www.hobbs.co.uk
HOUSE OF FLORA
mail@houseofflora.net
HOUSE OF FRASER 020 7963 2140
www.houseoffraser.co.uk
HUDSON JEANS FENWICK
020 7629 9161 www.ilovejeans.com
HUGO BOSS 020 7554 5700
HUIT www.figleaves.com
HUSH www.hush-uk2.com

I LOVE JEANS www.ilovejeans.com

J&M DAVIDSON 020 7313 9532
JAEGER 0845 051 0063
www.jaeger.co.uk
JAMES LOCK & CO 020 7930 8874
JENNERS 48 Princes Street,
Edinburgh EH2 0844 800 3725
www.houseoffraser.co.uk
JIGSAW 020 8392 5678
www.jigsaw-online.com
JIMMY CHOO 020 7823 1051
www.jimmychoo.com
JO GORDON www.jogordon.com
JOHN LEWIS 08456 049 049
www.johnlewis.com
JONATHAN ASTON 01277 232 301
www.tightsplease.co.uk
JOSEPH 020 7590 6200
www.joseph.co.uk
JOULES 0845 606 6871
www.joulesclothing.com
JOYCE RIDINGS
www.joyceridings.co.uk
JUICY COUTURE MATERNITY
www.JuicyCouture.com
BLOSSOM 020 7985 7480

*K*ANGOL 01946 818 350
www.kangol.com
KAREN MILLEN 0870 160 1830

KEW 020 8467 2001
www.kew-online.com
KURT GEIGER 0845 257 2571
www.kurtgeiger.com

*L*A PERLA 020 7291 0930
LA REDOUTE 0870 050 0455
www.laredoute.co.uk
LAND'S END www.landsend.co.uk
LANVIN MATCHES 020 7221 0255
www.matchesfashion.com
LAURA ASHLEY 0871 230 2301
www.lauraashley.com
LEPEL 0115 983 6000 www.lepel.com
LIBERTY 020 7734 1234
www.liberty.co.uk
LINKS OF LONDON 020 7730 3133
www.linksoflondon.com
LITTLEWOODS DIRECT 0845 757
3457 www.littlewoodsdirect.com
LIZA BRUCE 020 7235 8423
www.lizabruce.com
LK BENNETT 020 7491 3005
www.lkbennett.com
LL BEAN www.llbean.com
LOUIS VUITTON 020 7399 4050
LOVE FROM AUSTRALIA
www.lovefromaustralia.com

*M*ADE IN HEAVEN
www.ilovejeans.com
MADELEINE HAMILTON 020 7404
8484 www.madham.co.uk
MAIDENFORM www.figleaves.com
& www.rigbyandpeller.com
MANGO 020 7434 3694
www.mango.com
MANOLO BLAHNIK 020 7352 8622
MARGARET HOWELL 020 7009
9009 www.margarethowell.com
MARKS & SPENCER 0845 302 1234
www.marksandspencer.com
MARNI 020 7245 9520

MASSIMO DUTTI 020 7851 1280
MATTHEW WILLIAMSON
020 7629 6200
MAXMARA 020 518 8010
MEPHISTO www.mephisto.com
MINNETONKA
www.minnetonka.co.uk
MIRACLESUIT www.figleaves.com &
www.rigbyandpeller.com
MONSOON 0870 412 9000
www.monsoon.co.uk
MOSCHINO 020 7315 0555
MULBERRY 020 7491 3900
www.mulberry.com
MY PASHMINA
www.mypashmina.co.uk

N PEAL 020 7499 6485
www.npeal.com
NET-À-PORTER
www.net-a-porter.com
NEXT 0870 243 5435 www.next.co.uk
NICOLE FARHI 020 7499 8368
www.nicolefarhi.com
NOANOA 01225 428843
www.noanoa.com

*O*ASIS 01865 881 986
www.oasis-stores.com
OFFICE www.office.co.uk
ORLA KIELY 020 7240 4022
www.orlakiely.com

*P*AIGE PREMIUM DENIM
www.ilovejeans.com
PAPILLON BLUE 01530 245527
www.papillonbleu.com
PATRICIA www.rigbyandpeller.com
PAUL SMITH 020 7727 3553
www.paulsmith.co.uk
PEACOCKS 0115 965 8800
PHASE EIGHT 020 7471 4414
www.phase-eight.co.uk

PIED À TERRE 020 7380 3800
www.shoestudiogroup.com
PRADA 020 7647 5000
www.prada.com
PRETTY BALLERINAS
www.prettyballerinas.com
PRETTY POLLY
www.tightsplease.co.uk
PRIMA DONNA
www.rigbyandpeller.com
PRIMARK 0118 9606 300
www.primark.co.uk
PRINCIPLES 0870 122 8802
www.principles.co.uk
PURE COLLECTION
www.purecollection.com

R. SOLES 020 7351 5520
www.rsoles.com
RADLEY 08450 707080
www.radley.co.uk
RALPH LAUREN 020 7535 4600
REISS 020 7473 9600
www.reiss.co.uk
RIGBY & PELLER 0845 076 5545
www.rigbyandpeller.com
ROKIT 020 8801 8600 www.rokit.co.uk
RUPERT SANDERSON
0870 750 9181
www.rupertsanderson.com
RUSSELL & BROMLEY
020 7629 6903
www.russellandbromley.com

*S*AVILE ROW COMPANY
020 7432 9500 www.savillerowco.com
SELFRIDGES 0800 123 400
www.selfridges.com
SEVEN FOR ALL MANKIND Joseph
020 7590 6200 & www.ilovejeans.com
SISLEY 0845 389 9455
SJ PHILLIPS 020 7629 6261
www.sjphillips.com

SLACKS & CO 020 7352 8694
www.slacksandco.com
SLOGGI 01332 811732
www.justsloggi.co.uk
SOLANGE AZAGURY-PARTRIDGE
020 7792 0197
SPANX www.figleaves.com &
www.rigbyandpeller.com
SPLENDID HARVEY NICHOLS SW1
020 7235 5000
SELFRIDGES 0800 123 400
SPORTMAX 020 7518 8010
STELLA MCCARTNEY
020 7518 3100
www.stellamccartney.com
STEPHEN JONES 020 7242 0770
www.stephenjonesmillinery.com
SWEATY BETTY 0800 169 3889
www.sweatybetty.com

*T*ED BAKER 0845 130 4278
www.tedbaker.co.uk
THE CLASSIC BRETON SHIRT

www.bretonshirts.co.uk
THE NATURAL www.figleaves.com
THE SOCK SHOP
www.sockshop.co.uk
THE TIE RACK 020 8230 2333
www.tie-rack.co.uk
THE WHITE COMPANY
0870 900 9555
www.thewhitecompany.com
THEORY www.my-wardrobe.com
THOMAS PINK 020 7498 3882
www.thomaspink.com
TIFFANY & CO 25 Old Bond Street
W1 020 7499 4577 www.tiffany.com
T. M. LEWIN 0845 389 1898
www.tmlewin.co.uk
TOAST 0870 220 0460 www.toast.co.uk
TOD'S 020 7493 2237 www.tods.com
TOPSHOP 0845 121 4519
www.topshop.co.uk
TREASUREBOX
www.treasurebox.co.uk
TRIUMPH 01793 720300

www.triumph.com

*U*GG AUSTRALIA available from
Office nationwide
www.uggsdirect.co.uk
UNDER COVER
www.rigbyandpeller.com
UNIQLO www.uniqlo.co.uk
VIVIENNE WESTWOOD 020 7439
1109 www.viviennewestwood.com
VIYELLA 020 7200 2990
www.viyella.co.uk

*W*ALLIS 0870 830 0462
www.wallis-fashion.com
WAREHOUSE 0870 122 8813
www.warehousefashion.com
WHISTLES 0870 770 4301
www.whistles.co.uk
WOLFORD 020 7529 3000
www.wolfordboutiquelondon.com

*Z*ARA www.zara.com

BEAUTY

*A*MANDA LACEY 020 7584 0500
www.amandalacey.com
ARMANI (BEAUTY) Harvey Nichols
020 7201 8687
www.giorgioarmanibeauty.co.uk
AVEDA 0870 034 2380
www.aveda.co.uk
AVEENO 0845 601 5791
www.aveeno.co.uk
AVON 0845 601 4040
www.avonshop.co.uk

*B*ARBARA DALY FOR TESCO
0800 505 555
BENEFIT 0808 238 0230

BLISS 020 7590 6146
www.blisslondon.co.uk
BOBBI BROWN Space NK
Apothecary 020 8740 2085
www.spacenk.co.uk
BOOTS 0845 070 8090
BOURJOIS 0800 269 836
BUMBLE AND BUMBLE
020 7836 0818 www.spacenk.co.uk
BY TERRY Space NK Apothecary
020 8740 2085 www.spacenk.co.uk

*C*AUDALIE Space NK
Apothecary 020 8740 2085
www.spacenk.co.uk

CHANEL (BEAUTY) 020 7493 3836
www.chanel.com
CHANTECAILLE FENWICK London
W1 020 7629 9161
www.spacenk.co.uk
CLARINS 0800 036 3558
www.clarins.co.uk
CLINIQUE 01730 232566
www.clinique.co.uk
CRÈME DE LA MER Harrods London
SW1 020 7730 1234

*D*ANIEL GALVIN SALON
58–60 George Street, London W1
020 7486 8601

DDF Harvey Nichols
020 7235 5000
DECLÉOR 020 7313 8780
www.decleor.com
DERMALOGICA 0800 591 818
DIOR 020 7261 0261
DR ALKAITIS www.alkaitis.com
DR BRANDT
Space NK Apothecary
020 8740 2085 www.spacenk.co.uk
DR DENNIS GROSS
www.mdskincare.com
DR HAUSCHKA 01386 792642
www.drhauschka.co.uk
DREAS (PILATES) 020 7727 9963

*E*LEGANT NAILS 020 7792 2233
ELEMIS 01278 727830
www.elemis.com
ELIZABETH ARDEN
www.debenhams.com/beauty
ELEGANCE BEAUTY CLINIC 0207 792
2233 www.elegancebeautyclinic.com
ENVIRON www.firstforskincare.co.uk
ESTÉE LAUDER 0870 034 2566
EVE LOM Space NK Apothecary
020 8740 2085 www.spacenk.co.uk

*F*REDERIC FEKKAI www.spacenk.
co.uk & www.hqhair.com

*G*UERLAIN 01932 233887

*H*EADMASTERS SALON
11 Hanover Street, London W1
020 74081000

*J*AMES BROWN LONDON
selected Boots stores nationwide
www.boots.com
JANYCE WELCH (MASSAGE)
020 7373 9178
JEMMA KIDD selected Boots stores

nationwide www.jemmakidd.com
JOHN FRIEDA 020 7851 9800
www.johnfrieda.co.uk
JOHN FRIEDA SALON 4 Aldford
Street, London W1 020 7491 0840
JOHN LEWIS 0845 604 9049
www.johnlewis.com
JURLIQUE www.jurlique.co.uk

*K*AMINI 020 937 2411
www.kaminibeauty.com
KAY MONTANO www.kaymontano.com
KÉRASTASE available from Boots
stores nationwide www.boots.com
KIEHL'S Space NK Apothecary
020 8740 2085 www.spacenk.co.uk
KONJAC www.healthplus.co.uk

L'OCCITANE 020 7907 0301
www.loccitane.co.uk
L'ORÉAL www.lorealmakeup.co.uk
LA PRAIRIE Harrods, London SW1
020 7730 1234
LANCÔME www.lancome.co.uk
LAURA MERCIER Selfridges
020 7318 3378
LEAF & RUSHER Space NK
Apothecary 020 8740 2085
www.spacenk.co.uk
LIZ EARLE 01983 813913
www.lizearle.com

M LAB Harrods, London SW1
020 7730 1234
MAC 020 7534 9222
www.maccosmetics.co.uk
MARGARET DABBS 020 7487 5510
www.margaretdabbs.co.uk
MARY GREENWELL
www.marygreenwell.com
MASON PEARSON 020 7491 2613
www.masonpearson.com
MAX FACTOR available from Boots

stores nationwide www.boots.com
MICHAELJOHN SALON
25 Albemarle Street, London W1
020 7629 6969

*N*ARS Selfridges 0800 123 4000;
Space NK Apothecary 020 8740 2085
www.spacenk.co.uk
NEAL'S YARD REMEDIES 0845 262
3145 www.nealsyardremedies.com
NEUTROGENA 0545 601 5789
www.neutrogenauk.co.uk
NIVEA available from Boots stores
nationwide www.boots.com
NUDE 0800 634 4366
www.nudeskincare.com

*O*LAY available from Boots stores
nationwide www.boots.com
ORGANIC GLAM
www.theorganicpharmacy.com
ORGANIC PHARMACY
020 7351 2232
www.theorganicpharmacy.com
ORIGINS www.origins.co.uk

*P*HILIP KINGSLEY 020 7629 4050
PHILOSOPHY Selfridges 0800 123 400
POWER PLATE
http://uk.powerplate.com
PRESCRIPTIVES John Lewis & House
of Fraser nationwide www.johnlewis.
com; www.houseoffraser.co.uk

*R*EAL HAIR SALON 6–8 Cale St,
London, SW3 020 7589 0877
REN 0845 2255 600
www.renskincare.com
REVLON available from
Boots stores nationwide
www.boots.com
ROC available from Boots stores
nationwide www.boots.com

SALLY HANSEN 01276 674000
SHISEIDO Harrods 020 7730 1234
SHU UEMURA 020 7240 7635
SISLEY (BEAUTY) 020 7591 6380
SKINCEUTICALS 020 8997 8541
ST TROPEZ 0115 983 6363
STILA 020 7009 6290
www.spacenk.co.uk

TALIKA www.talika.com
THIS WORKS www.thisworks.com
TRISH MCEVOY Space NK
Apothecary 020 8740 2085
www.spacenk.co.uk

TWEEZERMAN www.skinstore.co.uk
VAISHALY www.vaishaly.com

VASELINE available from Boots stores
nationwide www.boots.com

WELEDA 0115 944 8222
www.weleda.co.uk

YVES SAINT LAURENT (BEAUTY)
01444 255700

BOUTIQUES

London

ANNA 126 Regents Park Road, NW1
020 7483 0411
BROWNS 23–27 South Molton St, W1
020 7514 0000
www.brownsfashion.com
FEATHERS 176 Westbourne Grove,
W11 020 7243 8800
A LA MODE 10 Symons St, SW3
020 7730 7180
MATCHES 60–64 Ledbury Rd, W11;
13 Hill St, Richmond; 34 High St,
Wimbledon, SW19 020 7221 0255
www.matchesfashion.com
JOSEPH 77 Fulham Road, SW3
020 7590 6200 www.joseph.co.uk

Nationwide

BERNARD OF ESHER 4–8 High
Street, Esher, KT10 9RT 01372 464604
www.bernardesher.co.uk
BISHOP PHILPOTT Castle Lodge,
10 Castle Street, Truro, TR1 3AF
01872 261750
BODY BASICS 79 Pontcanna Street,
Cardiff, CF11 9HS 029 2039 7025
www.body-basics.co.uk
BROWN THOMAS 88–95 Grafton
Street, Dublin, 2, Ireland +353 1 605
6666 www.brownthomas.com

CRICKET 10 Cavern Walks, Mathew
Street, Liverpool, L2 6RE 0151 227
4645 www.cricketliverpool.co.uk
CRUISE 180 Ingram St, Glasgow
0141 572 3232 www.cruiseclothing.co.uk
EMPORIO 33 Friar Street, Worcester,
WR1 2NA 01905 726643
FLANNELS 4 St Annes Place,
Manchester, M2 7LP 0161 832 5536;
55 King Street Manchester, M2 4LQ,
0161 839 7824; 68–78 Vicar Lane,
Leeds, LS1 7JH 0113 234 9977
www.flannelsfashion.com
GIULIO 24–32 King Street,
Cambridge, CB1 1LN, 01223 316100
JANE DAVIDSON 52 Thistle Street,
Edinburgh, EH2 1EN 0131 225 3280
www.janedavidson.co.uk
JEANNE PETITT 3 Bridge Street,
Hungerford, Berkshire RG17 OEH
01488 682472.
www.jeannepetitt.com
JULES B 91–93 Osborne Rd, Jes-
mond, Newcastle Upon Tyne, NE2
2AN 0191 281 7855 www.julesb.co.uk
L'AMICA 14 Post Office Road,
Bournemouth, BH1 1BA 01202 780033
MAGGIE & CO 7a Strand, Torquay,
TQ1 2AA 01803 292198

POLLYANNA 14–16 Market Hill,
Barnsley, S70 2QE 01226 291665
www.pollyanna.com
REPERTOIRE 104 Above Bar Street,
Southampton, SO14 7DT 023 8033 4001
RICHARD OLIVER 5 George Street,
St Albans, AL3 4ER 01727 859956
SELFRIDGES Birmingham Upper Mall
East, Bullring, Birmingham, B5 4BP
0800 123 400 www.selfridges.com
SQUARE 15 Old Bond Street, Bath
01225 464997 BA1 1BP
TESSUTI 14–20 Watergate Street,
Chester, CH1 2LA. 01244 312585
www.tessuti.co.uk
THE CLOTHES ROOM 1 Masham
Road, Harrogate, HG2 8QF
01423 889090
THE HAMBLEDON 10 The Square,
Winchester, Hampshire, SO23 9ES
01962 890055
www.thehambledon.com
YOUNG IDEAS St John Street,
Ashbourne, Derbyshire, DE6 1GP
01335 342095
www.youngideasfashion.com
ZOOMP 2 Jopps Lane, Aberdeen,
AB25 1BR 01224 642152
www.zoompclothing.co.uk

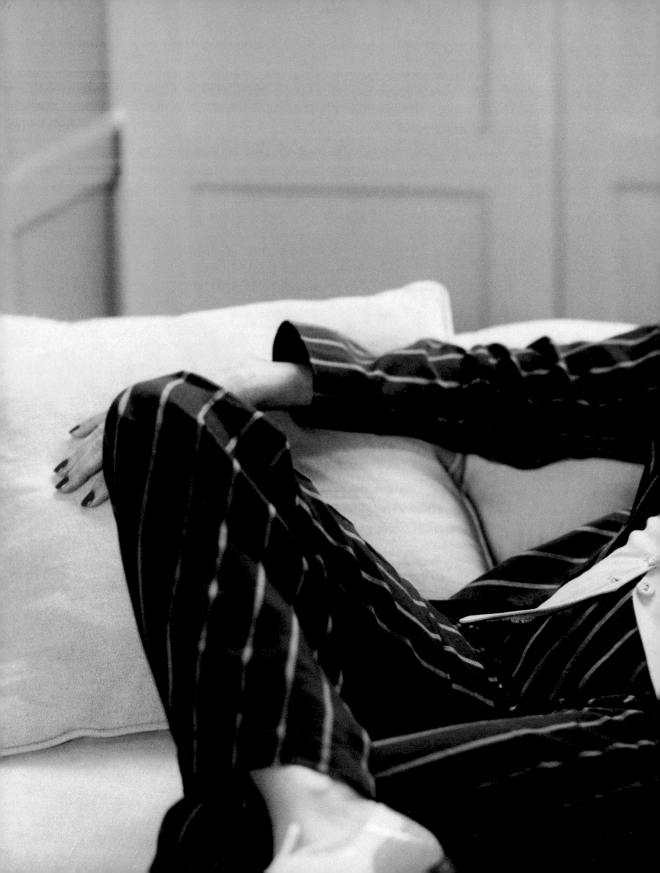

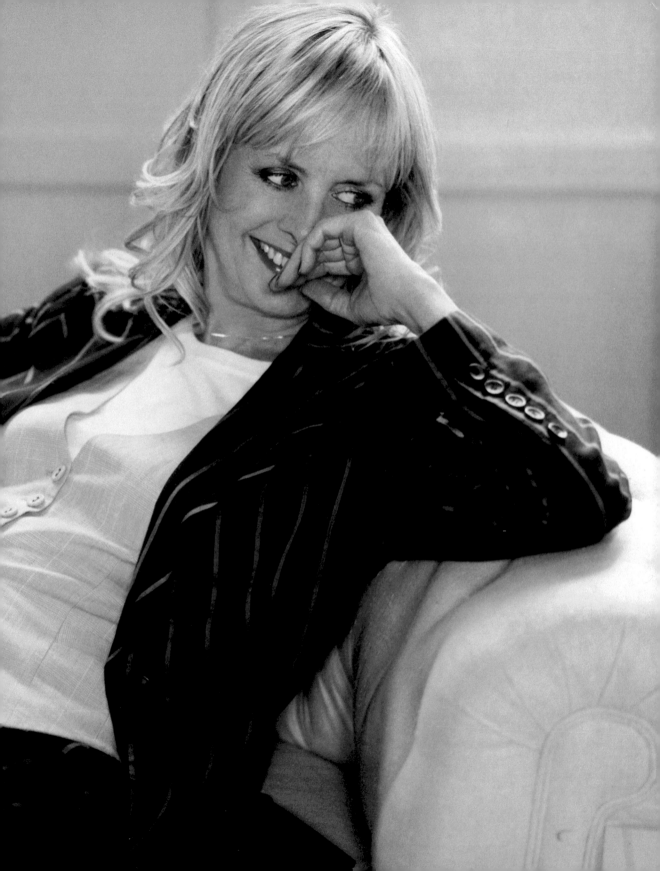

PICTURE CREDITS

with thanks

WITH SPECIAL THANKS TO:

- JENNY DYSON, thank you for your brilliant collaboration, intensely hard work and for all the laughter.

- CAROLINE MICHEL, the most stylish woman I know. Thank you for your unwavering faith. Your vision and guidance has changed my life.

- PENGUIN BOOKS
  LOUISE MOORE for her constant commitment, inspiration and guidance for this book.
  NIKKI DUPIN for her wonderful art direction.
  SARAH ROLLASON and CLARE POLLOCK and all the team at Penguin who have made this book a reality.

- BRIAN ARIS, you are the best! Thank you for all our wonderful shoots and your care and commitment always.

- SARAH MAINGOT, it was a pleasure to work with you and thank you for the results.

- TINA BERNING, thank you for your gorgeous illustrations. I adore them.

- BENOÎT AUDUREAU, for such beautiful still-life beauty shots.

- WILLIAM GARRETT, for my favourite M&S shot in the white suit.

- MATTHEW WADE, my favourite hairdresser – what would my hair do without you? Thank you also for the laughs.

- CHERYL PHELPS-GARDINER and CASSIE LOMAS, thank you for the beautiful make-up and the care you take on every session.

- TAMARA FULTON, thank you for all the hard work and the gorgeous styling.

- JULIETTE LEINWEBER, our wonderful PA. Thank you for your tireless hard work and keeping calm in all the madness!

- STUART ROSE and STEVE SHARP for the M&S campaign, which is so much fun. What visionaries and what great guys. I treasure our relationship and our friendship.

A big thank you to everyone who researched and gave advice for this book, without whom it would have been an impossible task.

- BARBARA DALY (who first did my make-up back in the 70s, and is a good friend) and KAY MONTANO for all their expert advice in the make-up section. Invaluable. Thank you also to MARY GREENWELL, KAMINI and ANTONIA WYATT. Your beauty insider knowledge has been second to none.

- DANIEL GALVIN and JOHN FRIEDA, old friends and brilliant in their field, thank you for your expert advice and input for the hair section. Also thank you to Josh Wood and Lester Baldwin for your tips on hair colour.

- Dermatologists DR DAVID COLBERT, DR FRANCES PRENNA JONES and DR NEIL WALKER. Thank you for demystifying the cosmetic surgery world!

with thanks

286

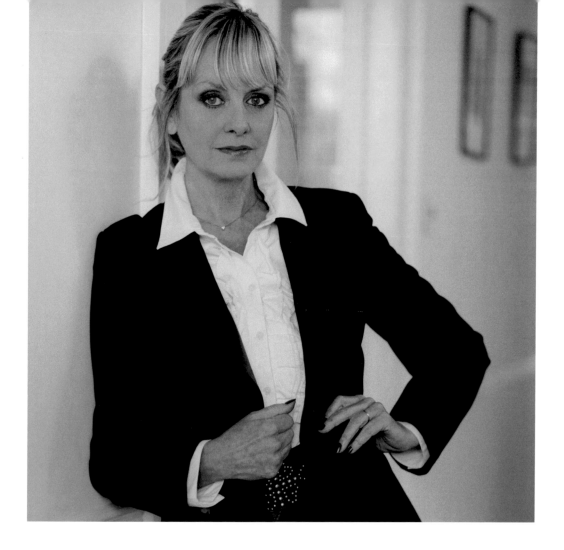

- Fabulous fashion designers CHRISTOPHER BAILEY, STELLA McCARTNEY, BETTY JACKSON and PAUL SMITH, you have all inspired many of the tips in this book. A big thank you all.

- Boutique owner JOAN BURSTEIN CBE, your style tips are faultless, your personal style an inspiration. MADELEINE HAMILTON and JUNE KENTON, thank you both for your input in the wardrobe and lingerie department.

- LAUREN HASSEY, thank you for being such a great research assistant. SAIREY STEMP, you are a shopping-directory genius! SOPHIE BAUDRAND, your input as a supremely gorgeous curvy girl was invaluable.

with thanks

287

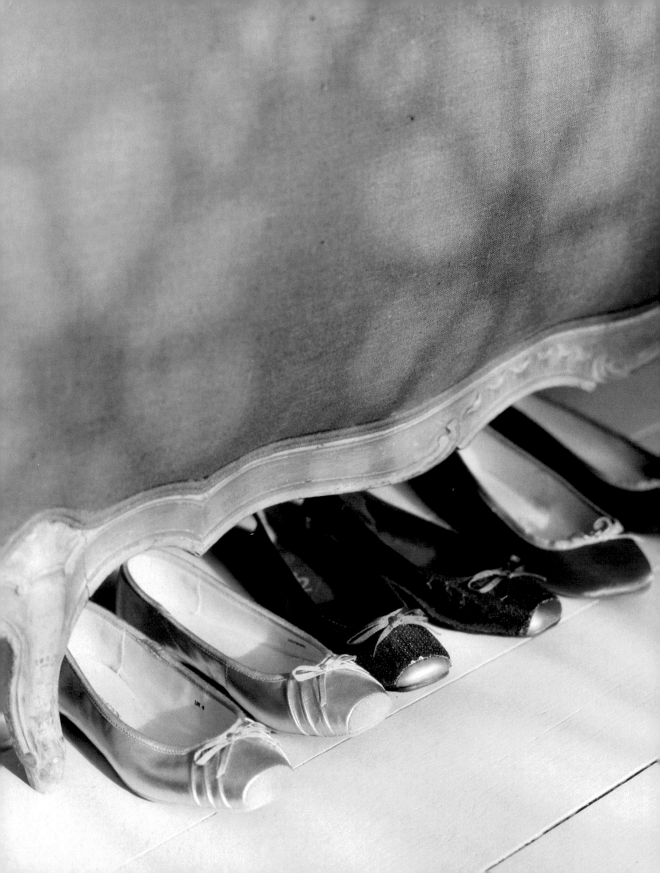